W9-API-178

Rachel Marie

Solution-Focused Therapy
with Children

Solution-Focused Therapy with Children

HARNESSING FAMILY STRENGTHS FOR SYSTEMIC CHANGE

Matthew D. Selekman

THE GUILFORD PRESS
New York   London

© 1997 The Guilford Press
A Division of Guilford Publications, Inc.
72 Spring Street, New York, NY 10012

Printed in the United States of America

This book is printed on acid-free paper.

Last digit is print number: 9 8 7 6 5 4 3 2

Library of Congress Cataloging-in-Publication Data

Selekman, Matthew D., 1957–
    Solution-focused therapy with children: harnessing family strengths for systemic change / Matthew D. Selekman.
        p.   cm.
    Includes bibliographical references and index.
    ISBN 1-57230-230-5
    1. Solution-focused therapy for children.   2. Family psychotherapy.   I. Title.
RJ505.S64S45   1997
618.92'8914—dc21   97-27
                                                                       CIP

Acknowledgments

There are several people I wish to acknowledge for greatly contributing to my professional development and the ideas discussed in this book. First and foremost, I want to thank Michele Weiner-Davis for showing me a variety of shortcuts for empowering clients and rapidly navigating them to "possibility land." I would like to thank Steve de Shazer and Insoo Kim Berg for providing me with several exceptional training experiences at the Brief Therapy Center in Milwaukee. From "down under," Michael White gets my undying appreciation for introducing me to the creative therapeutic pathway of externalizing problems. Finally, a special thanks to Tom Andersen, Harry Goolishian, and Harlene Anderson for exposing me to important postmodern therapy ideas, particularly, effective ways to collaborate with families that are therapy veterans and all the mental health professionals who are actively involved in those families' lives.

There are a few key people I would like to thank for paving the way for the creation of this book and its extra trimmings. From The Guilford Press, a big thanks to Kitty Moore, an excellent runner and superb editor, whose helpful editorial comments and guidance helped me put together a solid product, and to Anna Brackett, for her careful supervision of the production process. Thank you Don Efron for your helpful editorial comments. Laurie Callero, thank you for your patience with all of the revisions, tight deadlines, and your masterful typing abilities that helped me produce this manuscript. Finally, I would like to thank my loving and supportive wife Åsa, and Hanna, my little angel and other love, who constantly reminds me to make room for daily play and laughter.

Contents

CHAPTER 1

Expanding the Possibilities: An Integrative Solution-Focused Therapy Approach with Children

What moves men of genius, or rather what inspires
their work, is not new ideas, but their obsession with
the idea that what had already been said is still not
enough.
                                    –Eugène Delacroix

INTRODUCTION: MYTHS ABOUT CHILDREN AND THERAPY

President John F. Kennedy once said: "The greatest enemy of the truth
is not the lie—deliberate, contrived, and dishonest—but the myth—persistent, pervasive and unrealistic" (cited in Dawes, 1994, p. vii). Therapists hold many sacred cow beliefs about which methods and treatment
approaches are best suited for children. Child therapists argue that
family therapy approaches fail to attend adequately to the developmental concerns and intrapsychic conflicts of the child client. Family
therapists, on the other hand, maintain that the child's symptoms
indicate such family dysfunction as pathological structures or problem-
maintaining interaction patterns. Another widely held belief among
therapists is that treatment with children must be long term. In this
chapter, I first dispel some commonly held myths about children and
therapy and demonstrate why an integrative and flexible Solution-
Focused Therapy approach should be the model of choice for clinical
work with children and their families. I then present key findings from
research on resilient children which provides empirical support for this

claim. I follow with six ways I have expanded the basic Solution-Focused Therapy model to build in more therapeutic flexibility and options. Finally, the chapter concludes with a brief overview of the rest of the book.

"Young Children Should Be Excluded from Family Therapy Sessions"

It is commonplace for family therapists either to instruct parents to leave their youngest siblings at home with a babysitter or to place the youngest family members in a supervised play area in the office waiting room. Some family therapists believe that including young children in family sessions could be "psychologically harmful" to them or that they would be "highly disruptive" during the session. Others believe that young children will be unable to participate in session discussions or understand what is talked about because of their "developmental limitations."

However, there are several good reasons to include young children in family therapy sessions. Through young children's play and artwork we can gain access to family conflicts less accessible by verbal communication (Zilbach, Bergel, & Gass, 1972). Often, children's play and artwork are metaphors for how they view themselves and significant relationships in their families. Eliciting feedback from the parents and older siblings of the young child about his or her play and artwork can open up avenues for challenging outmoded family beliefs and unhelpful parent–child interactions. Keith and Whitaker (1994) contend that "play is the medium for expanding the family's reality" (p. 194). Young children inject spontaneity and playfulness into family sessions. The young child can serve as a co-therapist in teaching his or her parents how to play again. Finally, young children's presence in family sessions affords the opportunity for the therapist to model positive and nurturing interactions for the parents.

"Traumatized Children Will Grow Up to Be Emotionally Flawed Adults"

Undoubtedly, some children who have been traumatized by various forms of parental abuse or who have experienced painful losses produce emotional scars that haunt them for the rest of their lives. The trauma literature is filled with examples about the deleterious effects of traumatic events on a child's individual and interpersonal functioning. Yet, over the past few decades little discussion in this literature about the growing body of resiliency research has identified children who experienced multiple traumatic events in their lives and managed to grow up to be well-functioning adults. As Garmezy (1991) has pointed out, the resilient individual is characterized by "the maintenance of competent functioning despite an interfering emotionality" (p. 416). In commenting on some widely held beliefs in the sex abuse treatment field, Trepper and Barrett (1989) say:

> The belief that sexual abuse will lead to severe emotional problems has been the cornerstone of all therapy. . . . Most therapists probably believe this without hesitation, and probably justify some of their most intrusive therapeutic measures on it. The research on the long-term effects of child sexual abuse has been quite mixed, however. (p. 11)

Garmezy (1993) also argues that there are not enough empirically based longitudinal studies of long-term outcomes of child abuse cases to support the widely held belief that an abused child will grow up to become an adult abuser.

Here I present two major studies conducted with trauma survivors who "beat the odds" and grew up to be well-functioning adults.

Moskovitz (1983) conducted an exploratory study with a group of Holocaust survivors to determine how they coped with their hellish experiences in the Nazi concentration camps during World War II. None of her subjects succumbed to suicide attempts, alcohol or drug abuse, or psychiatric disorders. She noted that "their hardiness of spirit and their quiet dignity are part of this persistent endurance" (p. 233). Moskovitz (1983) further added:

> Despite the severest deprivation in early childhood, these people are neither living greedy, me-first style of life, nor are they seeking gain at the expense of others. None express the idea that the world owes them a living for all they have suffered. On the contrary, most of their lives are marked by a compassion for others. (p. 233)

Festinger (1983) followed 277 children in New York City who were placed in foster care early in childhood until young adulthood. Many of these children were emotionally and physically abused, were abandoned, had a mentally ill or drug-addicted parent, or lost a parent through death. Approximately 69% of her sample had been to three to four foster homes or institutions as young children. When comparing all 277 of these young adults to a sample of subjects from a national survey conducted by the Institute of Social Research at the University of Michigan, she discovered the following: Although the foster care subjects showed lower scholastic achievements, their employment rates, health and symptoms status, and personal evaluations of their feelings, future hopes, and current sense of happiness were similar. Festinger (1983) noted that her foster care subjects were generous contributors to the study and exhibited a willingness and openness to discuss their lives in the hope that it would help others.

What the previous studies did not mention was that each of the subjects possessed a unique set of protective factors that helped insulate them from the onslaught of multiple stressors and adverse life events throughout their childhoods. Without these protective factors, such as social competence and nurturing support systems (Garmezy, 1994), the research subjects' adult lives might have turned out differently. Later in this chapter, I discuss further the role of protective factors in the adaptation process, as well as how resiliency research can inform our clinical practices.

When working with children who were traumatized, we need to empower them to become masters of their own lives. We can do this by conveying an optimistic attitude, capitalizing on their competency areas, respecting their defenses, and giving them room to tell their painful stories when, or if, they are ready to do so. As therapists, we need to be sensitive to the fact that our theoretical maps and the way we interact with our clients determine what we see. If we operate from a deficit-oriented model, we inevitably see deficits and become expert repairmen and -women. By capitalizing on our young clients' strengths and resources and what is "going right" in their present lives, we can help these children create their own positive self-fulfilling prophecies.

"Children Should Be Seen and Not Heard in the Treatment Planning and Problem-Solving Process"

More often than not, children are not given a voice in their own treatment or school educational planning. Typically, when a family presents for therapy, the parents' goals take precedence as the focus for treatment without any exploration with the child about what his or her goals or expectations might be. We see this a great deal in child abuse cases. With most child abuse cases, the treating therapist, the child protective worker, and other involved representatives from larger systems determine the treatment goals and treatment plan for the child and the family. Often at multidisciplinary school staffings, children are excluded when an individual educational plan is being developed for them, and, if they are lucky, they will be invited in at the end of the meeting to hear what direction their school year will take in terms of special services or placement. Not only do the children have no input in the final individual educational plan, but they have no opportunity to give any feedback on the school psychologist's case study evaluation results, which are typically discussed in the multidisciplinary staffing.

When working with children and their families, I invite the child to share his or her goals and expectations. Some children may have a goal for their parents (e.g., to "yell" less). I believe it is possible to attend simultaneously to the parents' and child's goals. Also, I explore whether the children are having any difficulties with siblings or specific teachers with whom they would like me to intervene. To help take the focus off the identified child client being labeled by the parents and others as the "bad kid," I recommend to the parents, as an experiment, to carefully observe for 1 week the angelic "good kid's" behavior when he or she is around the identified client. Frequently, parents discover that their angelic child is a master at pushing their so-called problem child's buttons. This intervention helps to show the interactional component of the presenting problem and to challenge the parents' beliefs that the problem lies with one child. Finally, whenever possible, I try to include the child in any collaborative meetings with school personnel and with other involved representatives from larger systems.

In a recent exploratory study with children who had received family therapy, the researchers discovered from the children themselves that the children expected to be included in family sessions and to have a voice in discussions and participate in the problem-solving process. The children also appreciated therapists who displayed warmth and concern toward them (Stith, Rosen, McCollum, Coleman, & Herman, 1996). Research of this kind helps provide empirical support for the importance of giving children a voice in their own treatment.

"Severe and Chronic Child Behavioral Difficulties Will Require Big and Complex Solutions"

In an earlier work (Selekman, 1993), I discussed the evolutionary process of how cases become "difficult." Typically, the so-called difficult case keeps receiving "more of the same" treatment variety (Watzlawick, Weakland, & Fisch, 1974), and the child's and family's problems become further compounded and exacerbated while on the treatment circuit, collecting a variety of labels out of the DSM-IV (the fourth edition of the *Diagnostic and Statistical Manual of Mental Disor-*

ders; American Psychiatric Association, 1994). In commenting on the labeling process, Wittgenstein (1980) warned us against unwarranted completion in our descriptions of essentially incomplete human activities still in progress: "If you complete it, you falsify it" (p. 257). In other words, once a child has been labeled with a particular problem or disorder, there will be no other way of thinking about this child—past, present, and future.

When working with children and families that have experienced multiple treatment failures, it behooves us to explore with them what they disliked about former therapists, so as to avoid making the same kind of mistakes. I like to empower these families by placing them in the expert position and asking them the following questions:

> "You have seen a lot of therapists before me, what did they miss with your situation?"

> "On your way to my office, did you think about all of the possible ways I could screw up your case?" (with clients being labeled "noncompliant")

> "What didn't you like with former therapists, so I don't make the same mistakes?"

> "If I were to work with another family just like yours, what advice would you give me to help that family out?"

> "If you were to work with the most perfect therapist what would he or she do that you would find to be most helpful?"

It is also helpful with so-called professional families to negotiate small and solvable goals, with the family deciding what they want to work on changing first. With some of these families, past therapists' goals may have driven the treatment: either they had no idea what their clients' goals were, or the clients' goals were too monolithic, such as trying to change many symptoms-bearers simultaneously. When the latter is the case, I find it most useful to break up the family and work with family subsystems or individuals (Selekman, 1993).

"The Therapist Is More of an Expert on Parenting Than the Child's Parents"

Many therapists adopt a privileged, expert position with the parents and children with whom they work. It is hard not to fall into this trap.

The more specialized training and knowledge we secure in a particular therapy approach, the more overconfident we become in our therapeutic abilities and with our models of choice. As Palmarini (1994) warns: "We need to be wary of our overconfidence which tends to be at its greatest in our own area of expertise and where it can do the most damage" (p. 119). There are many popular parenting models that therapists have adopted as their road maps for parent training, such as the PET (Gordon, 1970) and STEP (Dinkmeyer & McKay, 1989) models. Some child therapists believe that they are better equipped than the child's parents to provide their young clients with missing "selfobject functions" (Kohut, 1971) or to help them resolve their intrapsychic conflicts. The same is true with play therapy. The parents arc rarely included in the child's play or art activities.

It is my contention that our main expertise as therapists should be in eliciting the parents' expertise. Any past successes that parents have had at resolving other behavioral difficulties can be used as models for present and future successes. In all problematic parenting situations, there are times when the parents are managing their children's behaviors well and are enjoying their tough jobs. Like a Columbo or Miss Marple detective, we need to inquire about what specifically parents are doing during those nonproblem times that is working for them. These key parental problem-solving and coping strategies can serve as building blocks in the solution-construction process. Similarly, taking the time in the first family session to find out from parents what their strengths and talents are in their work roles can provide therapists with valuable information that they can utilize in developing potential solution strategies. Finally, why not include parents in the child's in-session play and art therapy activities. Doing so can help reduce family stress, improve family communications, and teach parents and children fun ways to solve conflicts and problems.

SUPERKIDS: HOW RESILIENCY RESEARCH CAN INFORM OUR CLINICAL PRACTICES

In speaking out against the "Diseasing of America" (Peele, 1989) trend in the media and in the world of mental health care, Wolin (Wolin, O'Hanlon, & Hoffman, 1995) has argued: "We need a list of strengths as powerful and as validating as the florid vocabulary of diseases found in DSM-IV to combat our national obsession with pathology" (p. 24). Wolin (Wolin & Wolin, 1993) and a group of psychologists and psychiatrists have been studying high-risk children's psychosocial competencies and resourcefulness over the past two decades. When faced with adversity and stressful life events, these researchers found that many of the children in their studies consistently "bounced back" quickly and "beat the odds" (Anthony & Cohler, 1987; Haggerty, Sherrod, Garmezy, & Rutter, 1994; Wolin & Wolin, 1993).

I now provide an overview of three of the key protective factors found in these researchers' studies (see Table 1.1) with high-risk children reared in poverty and high-stress family environments characterized by violence, parental alcoholism and substance abuse, divorce, and parental mental illness. This overview is followed by a discussion of how to develop, enhance, and utilize these key protective factors in our therapeutic work with children and their families.

TABLE 1.1. Key Protective Factors of Resilient Children

Individual factors	Family factors	Extrafamilial support factors
Optimistic explanatory style	Caring and supportive parents	Nurturing support system (relatives, friends, teachers, neighbors, and inspirational significant others)
Good sense of humor	Strong parent–child relationships	
Self-efficacy		
Strong social skills	Low levels of family conflict	Church involvement
Cognitive competence	Optimistic parenting explanatory styles	Successful school experiences
Good-natured temperament		
Pronounced self-sufficiency		
Robustness		
Sense of coherence		
Perseverance		
Involvement in creative activities		
Intelligence		
Strong problem-solving skills		
Good management of emotions		
Keen sense of self-awareness		

Effective and Creative Problem-Solvers

One of the most frequent findings in all the reviewed studies with high-risk children was that these children had strong problem-solving abilities. These children were described as "resourceful," "creative," and "acting" rather than "reacting" to the problems and crises they faced (Anthony, 1987; Garmezy, 1981, 1994; Masten & Garmezy, 1985; Masten, Best, & Garmezy, 1990; Werner, 1987a, 1987b; Werner & Smith, 1982, 1992; Wolin & Wolin, 1993). Many of these children viewed problems as challenges they were confidently prepared to face and master—a finding in studies on children deemed optimistic (Diener & Dweck, 1978; Dweck, 1975; Seligman, 1995). As a way of coping with crises and problems, some of these children would seek solace by going to church, spending time with a close friend or an inspirational other, or engaging in sports or other recreational activities (Anthony, 1984, 1987; Masten et al., 1990; Wolin & Wolin, 1993).

Anthony (1987) has identified two types of cognitive competency areas displayed by resilient children: *constructive competence* and *creative competence*. Constructive competence is characterized by a practical and concrete approach to tasks and problem solving. These children are independent and self-confident when carrying out tasks. Creative competence is demonstrated by the child's ability to move from practical ways of solving problems to more abstract and novel ways of problem solving.

In applying this important protective factor to clinical practice, in the initial family assessment session I explore with the child and his or her parents what the identified child client has done both in the past and in the present to resolve problems or better cope with them. I have some children visualize memorable successful problem-solving experiences and utilize these movies of success to empower them to resolve their presenting problems. It is also helpful to find out from the parents what they have done successfully in the past to help the child better cope with life stressors and resolve difficulties. These successful problem-solving strategies can be used in the current problem area. Sometimes I have a child and his or her family create a Victory Box. They can record on paper personal triumphs, achievements, and problem-solving efforts in school, at home, in sports events, at work, or with the creative arts and place their written documentation of their personal victories in the box. The Victory Box serves as a clearinghouse for blueprints of success and mastery for the child and his or her family.

If the child is presented by the parents and referring person as having "poor problem-solving abilities," I still explore with the child and his or her parents what interests, talents, and skills the identified child client possesses that I can use in this problem area. For example, if the child has a strong interest in science and performs well academically in this subject area, I have the child identify his or her most favorite scientists and inventors and discuss how they solved problems. I then have the child use some of these scientists' and inventors' unique problem-solving strategies to experiment with the problems he or she faces. Role playing the child's problem situation can also be useful as a skill-building method for teaching the child new problem-solving strategies. However, it is even more effective to include the identified child client's "pal" in the role-play activity. The friend may be able to offer and model for the child client more effective problem-solving strategies than the therapist could provide.

Strong Social Skills

Another important protective factor for resilient children is their strong social skills. Many of the researchers who studied these high-risk children were struck by the children's knack for establishing and maintaining relationships with peers, neighbors, clergy, and other adults. Not only were these children naturals at establishing support systems for themselves, but they could reach out with ease to a friend, parent, or other adult for support in time of crisis (Anthony, 1984, 1987; Garmezy, 1994; Masten et al., 1990; Kauffman, Grunebaum, Cohler, & Gamer, 1979; Wolin & Wolin, 1993). Their solid assertiveness skills were an important strength that helped shield them from becoming clinically depressed (Garmezy, 1981, 1994; Masten et al., 1990; Masten & Garmezy, 1985; Seligman, 1995). In his St. Louis Risk Research Project with inner-city African American children, Anthony (1984, 1987) found that many of these children sought out and established a relationship with a charismatic or inspirational person in their communities who "turned them on," sustained them, and continued to have long-lasting effects on them throughout their lives.

Most of the researchers observed that the resilient children's social competence proved to be self-esteem building for them and contributed to their success in school (Garmezy, 1994; Masten et al., 1990; Werner & Smith, 1982, 1992). Most of the emotional needs for some of the resilient children in these studies were met through their social involvement with concerned neighbors, teachers, clergy, and friends' parents.

Clinically speaking, we can capitalize on a child's strong social skills by incorporating their friend, inspirational other, and other concerned adults in the treatment process as consultants. These consultants may offer the therapist, the child, and his or her parents some useful ideas about how to solve the presenting problem and better cope with life stressors. For children who have poor social skills, we can use role playing to teach assertiveness skills. The identified child client's friend can be used as a resource person when using the role-play strategy.

Supportive and Responsible Caretakers

Most of the research on high-risk children challenges the widely held belief among social scientists and mental health professionals that these children lack a caring and responsible adult in their lives. In fact, many of the studies reviewed indicated that these children received considerable attention from responsible caretakers in their early years of development and throughout their childhoods. Even children who had a mentally ill or alcoholic or drug-impaired parent described times when their parent was very loving, and supportive and met their needs (Anthony, 1987; Bleuler, 1978; Kauffman et al., 1979; Wolin & Wolin, 1993). In some cases, a relative, an adult friend of the family, or the nonsymptomatic parent assumed the main caretaker role for the child. Kauffman et al. (1979) observed in their study that nonsymptomatic parents played a critical role in helping their at-risk children function and cope well with family stressors. Many of the supportive and responsible caretaking adults in the studies maintained optimistic parental explanatory styles (Seligman, 1995). These parental figures displayed unconditional positive regard, were flexible, modeled the importance of being optimistic when faced with life's struggles, and taught their children how to separate one isolated failure from others and to challenge their pessimistic views (Anthony, 1987; Bleuler, 1978; Garmezy, 1994; Kauffman et al., 1979; Wolin & Wolin, 1993).

In the clinical arena, this research finding provides empirical support for educating parents about the importance of adopting an optimistic parenting style and demonstrates how such education can greatly influence their children's optimism and behavior when they are faced with stressful life events. In fact, Seligman (1995) has found in his research that parental optimism is a key protective factor for children at risk for becoming clinically depressed. Giving parents observation tasks to keep track of what the child does that is "right" and responsible, asking questions about past successes, and having the parents visualize positive treatment outcomes can help create a therapeutic climate of optimism for the child and his or her family. For families that tend to be overly focused on the negative, I assign the construction of a Compliment Box. On a daily basis, each family member is responsible for writing on a piece of paper a compliment for another family member and placing it in the box. At dinner time, a designated family member can read off the compliments. The Compliment Box system helps to reduce blaming and negativity in the family and creates a more positive atmosphere in the home. Finally, grandparents and other significant caretaking adults in the child's life can be utilized as expert consultants to both the therapist and the parents.

In spite of being raised in high-risk family and social environments, the good news is that children can and do survive adverse life experiences. Some children are born naturally resilient; others are quite skilled at creating nurturing support systems for themselves outside their families. The research on resilient children has uncovered many ways that we, as therapists, can help strengthen family relationships and help children find strength and success beyond their families.

ADAPTING THE SOLUTION-FOCUSED THERAPY MODEL FOR CHILDREN

Like all therapy models, the basic Solution-Focused Brief Therapy approach has its limitations with certain types of child cases, even after exhausting all the therapeutic options within the model. Before discussing three clinical case situations in which it may be necessary to expand the basic model and integrate and apply therapeutic ideas from individual and other family therapy approaches, I discuss some of the limitations of the Solution-Focused Brief Therapy approach with children.

To begin with, the Solution-Focused Brief Therapy approach is a "talk therapy," which does not mesh well with young children's natural tendencies to express themselves best through nonverbal means (e.g., play and art activities). Young children are not capable of cognitively understanding such abstract concepts as "miracles" and "goals." The Solution-Focused questions in general may be incomprehensible or too difficult to grasp for some children, even after the therapist concretizes the wording of the questions. Many Solution-Focused therapists believe that simply altering parental beliefs and interactions with the child will lead to the latter's changing. This assumption is based on the systems concept of *wholism*; that is, if you change one part of the family system, the other members of the family will change as well (de Shazer, 1985). Most Solution-Focused therapists, and family therapists for that matter, would not consider the idea that children can serve as the catalyst for changing their parents' and family interactions through the use of family play and art activities. De Shazer (1988) has pointed out that therapists should draw from the set of "all known tasks" once they have exhausted all the standard therapeutic tasks typically used within the basic Solution-Focused model. What he does not provide for the reader, however, are recommended therapeutic tasks and strategies from other therapy approaches that may be useful with particular types of children's problems and clinical case situations.

At this point, I present three case situations in which I found it helpful to expand the basic Solution-Focused model and to be more therapeutically flexible:

1. The parents change their ways of viewing and interacting with the identified child client; however, the child remains symptomatic.

2. The parents' treatment goals are achieved, but the changes in the identified child client are not perceived by them as "newsworthy"; thus, their outmoded beliefs about the child and their situation remain intact.

3. There are multiple helping professionals involved with the case, many of whom are highly pessimistic about the identified child client and his or her family's ability to change.

By expanding the basic Solution-Focused Brief Therapy model and being therapeutically flexible, each of these clinical case situations can be adequately managed. In the first case scenario, family play and art therapy tasks, visualization techniques, and cognitive skills training open the door to the child's inner world and help remove constraints or blocks in affective or cognitive areas of functioning which may be preventing symptom alleviation. Some children in such cases, depending on their age and the results of a child psychiatrist's evaluation, may benefit from a low dosage of medication.

In the second case scenario, there may be family secrets, unresolved traumas and losses, or other family concerns not being talked about, or the therapist has blocked family members from sharing their long, problem-saturated stories by overemphasizing the positive in sessions. Two common parental concerns I have experienced in these types of child case situations is my failure to confirm and accept the DSM-IV label to which they are wedded or my failure to take their child's chronic presenting problems "seriously enough." By saying the therapist is not taking their child's presenting problems seriously enough, the parents may be trying to express that they want the therapist to work with their child individually more on a long-term basis. Open-ended conversational questions (Anderson & Goolishian, 1988b; Selekman, 1993) can be used to give family members ample space to share their concerns and the "not yet said," such as disclosing a family secret or a painful life event. Another therapeutic option in this case scenario would be to use a "reflecting team" (Andersen, 1991, 1995) to offer the family a multiplicity of views on their family concerns and difficulties. This can help loosen up fixed family beliefs and open up space for the family members to view their situation differently.

Finally, in the third case scenario, a therapist hosting a family–multiple helper collaborative meeting or attending a multidisciplinary school staffing may come across as too optimistic or overzealous about reporting the positives in a chronic child case, and group conversations and input from the more pessimistic helpers attending these meetings may be shut down. Therefore, when hosting or attending such meetings, therapists, no matter what their theoretical persuasion, can adopt the Buddhist stance of "don't know mind," which is a true "both/and" perspective (Selekman, 1993). As the hosting therapist, he or she must be able to suspend his or her assumptions about the helpers' and family's concerns, to learn to view them as assumptions and not facts, and to hold them in front of the group for all to see (Isaacs, 1993). Similar to attending to the concerns of a pessimistic family member, the therapist needs to create a safe space for the pessimistic helpers to voice their concerns about the case. It is important to remember that there are many ways to view a child or family's presenting problems and that consensus in the family–multiple helper collaborative meetings or among school staff is not required in order to have effective group problem solving and to generate new family narratives.

A final reason for expanding the basic Solution-Focused Brief Therapy model and utilizing a more integrative approach is that such expansion increases our repertoire of interpretation schemes and offers us a broader range of therapeutic options when intervening with children and their families. Research also indicates that there is compelling evidence for the effectiveness of integrative family therapy approaches for children with behavioral problems (Lebow & Gurman, 1996).

THE EVOLUTION OF AN INTEGRATIVE SOLUTION-FOCUSED BRIEF THERAPY APPROACH FOR CHILDREN

In this section, I present the six major therapeutic components of the integrative Solution-Focused Brief Therapy model. I discuss each therapeutic component and how it improves the basic Solution-Focused Brief Therapy approach by providing more therapeutic options within the model. Case examples are provided.

Finding the "Right" Problem

The famous philosopher and educator John Dewey believed that any problem that is well-defined is half-solved (Parnes, 1992). For a number of reasons (e.g., managed health care), there is a strong tendency among therapists to try to find the quick solution for their clients' problems without taking the time to determine collaboratively with the clients what the "real" or "right" problem is. Leading proponents of the basic Solution-Focused Brief Therapy model argue that therapists do not need to know a great deal about their clients' problems to solve them and that therapists should avoid at all costs engaging in "problem talk" (Berg & de Shazer, 1991) with their clients. However, going with an ill-defined client problem will make any constructed or selected solution ineffective in the long run. Finding the right client problem is equivalent to finding the right solution for resolving it. Problems and solutions are close relatives and do not always need to be separated for effective problem solving (Van Gundy, 1988).

A number of studies have provided empirical support for the importance of problem defining in creative problem solving (Csikszentmihalyi & Getzels, 1970; Getzels & Csikszentmihalyi, 1975, 1976a, 1976b; Moore, 1985; Rokeach, 1950). In his study, Rokeach (1950) found that deferred judgment or giving oneself more time to explore a problem situation tends to decrease rigidity in solution finding. Csikszentmihalyi and Getzels (1970) investigated the relationship between problem defining and artistic creativity. The artists in the study were instructed to produce a drawing using a variety of objects that had been placed on a table in front of them. A panel of well-known artists and art critics judged the drawings. The results of the study suggested that the artists who approached the art task with no set problem in mind and who avoided using any predetermined artistic patterns or formulas produced more original and creative drawings than did those artists who began with a predetermined approach. Interestingly, the highly rated artists spent considerably more time manipulating the objects on the table. Two important findings can be extracted from this study that can inform our clinical practices: (1) Take the time to find the right problem in order to understand where to begin with the family, and (2) avoid using a predetermined formula for problem solving.

Families that have been oppressed by their problems for a long time and have experienced multiple treatment failures may feel slighted and unheard when a therapist fails to give them ample space to share their long, problem-saturated stories. According to Anderson (1996), "Understanding too quickly cuts a client's story short and risks eliciting the story that a therapist wants to hear, rather than the story a client wants to tell" (p. 202). Fraser (1995) argues that unless we take the time to elicit from families their attempted solutions and views of the problem, we will have no idea when their problems are really solved. The first case helps illustrate the importance of both taking the time to collaboratively determine with the family the right problem to work on first and making room for their story about the problem situation.

> Ellen, 10 years old, was brought in for therapy by her mother for attention-deficit disorder (ADD), "stealing," "lying," "doing poorly" in school, "fighting" with her siblings, and "breaking" her mother's "rules." According to her mother, Ellen had been sexually molested when she was 6 years old by an uncle. Sensing the mother's strong feelings of hopelessness and despair about being able to help her daughter, I gave her plenty of room to share her problem-saturated story. I also gathered detailed information about her attempted solutions, particularly what past therapists had tried to do with Ellen and her mother that the mother did not find helpful. After receiving ample space to ventilate her frustration about former therapists and the problem situation, the mother became much more receptive to clarifying with me what she perceived as the right problem to work on first. She believed that Ellen engaged in all these difficult behaviors because of "the trauma" of Ellen's being sexually molested at the age of 6. The stealing behavior in particular began at this time, which was the mother's "greatest source of irritation." The mother agreed with me that it would be too monolithic a task to try to change all of Ellen's behaviors at once. For both the mother and Ellen, the right problem to work on changing first was the stealing behavior.

After hearing the mother's frustrations with past therapists and Ellen's chronic behavior problems, it was clear to me that the mother would have felt slighted and would have viewed me as being like all the other overzealous therapists she had seen in the past if I had moved too quickly to talk about exceptions or asked the miracle question (de Shazer, 1988; see Chapter 2, this volume). By giving the mother ample space to share her long, problem-saturated story without any therapeutic editing, I was in a much better place to define the problem to work on first. Future therapy sessions were focused on systematically stabilizing each of Ellen's behavior problems and collaborating with concerned school personnel.

Use of Family Play and Art Therapy Strategies

For decades, child and family therapists have vigorously debated which treatment modality is best suited for children. Child therapists would argue that the child's behavioral and emotional difficulties are caused by faulty parenting that results in intrapsychic conflicts, developmental arrests, or possible psychic deficits. Through the use of art and play therapy methods, a child therapist provides a safe climate for children to play out their conflicts and uses his or her therapeutic relationship with the child to try to heal the psychic deficits (Kohut, 1971). The parents are typically seen separately or by another therapist. Family therapists would argue that the child's problems should be viewed through a broader lens. The "problem" child's symptoms may serve a function in the family (Haley, 1987; Madanes, 1981) and may be on account of structural problems in the family (Minuchin, 1974), perpetuated by problem-maintaining parental attempted solutions (Watzlawick et al., 1974), and maintained by constraining beliefs and dominant oppressive stories (White & Epston, 1990). Most family therapists would actively involve the parents in the treatment process. Depending on the model being used, the family therapist focuses most of his or her attention on changing outmoded beliefs about the child and altering patterns of behavior that may be maintaining the problems. Some family therapists focus most of their therapeutic attention on changing the parents and spend very little time interacting with the child alone.

It is my contention that both the individual and the family therapy perspectives offer therapeutic techniques that complement one another, as long as what the therapist chooses to do therapeutically is purposive and in line with the family's goals. In general, children, and particularly young children, like to play and rarely respond well to talk therapies alone. Sometimes the parents' ways of viewing and interacting with the child change but the child remains symptomatic. One therapeutic option in such cases is to use art and play therapy techniques. However, rather than seeing children alone to perform these tasks, I have found it most advantageous to include the parents as both participants and observers in the art and play therapy activities.

Wachtel (1994) and Gil (1994) use a similar format in their clinical work with children and their families. With some cases, it might be a novel experience for both the child and the parents to play with one another or to create a family picture together. Family play and art therapy tasks can take the sting out of presenting problems, reduce stress levels, loosen up fixed beliefs about the problem, and alter the family dance in which the problem is embedded. The therapist also gains access to destructive problem interactions and family conflicts which he or she can address directly in a relaxed context in which anything is possible. Sometimes children's art creations can serve as the catalyst for changing and healing their parents. The following case example illustrates this point.

> Sandra, 6 years old, was brought for therapy by her parents, Bill and Evelyn, who were separated after their second marriage to each other. The couple separated after Bill began slapping and pushing Evelyn around when they got into an argument. Both parents were quick to point out their long history of arguing and getting physical with one another.
>
> Sandra lived with her mother and 10-month-old brother, Evan. Despite the parents' difficulties, they were both concerned about Sandra's passivity and wondered whether she was "depressed." Sandra appeared to be very shy and timid. Efforts to engage her went nowhere until I asked her to draw a picture of her family. The parents were quite shocked and cried when they saw Sandra's drawing. Sandra drew a picture of her family floating in air around the interior of the house; she placed herself outside the front door. She drew very thick lines around the house and had the front door closed.
>
> Seeing this drawing proved to be an eye-opening and emotional experience for the parents. Sandra was also able to talk about how she did not feel "safe" when her parents were together. The child protection and local police departments had a history of involvement with this case and were still involved as a result of domestic disputes. Despite all the chaos in the home, the children were never physically harmed. By the end of the session, the

parents were open to working on their problems with anger management, conflict resolution, and violent behavior. We established a no-violence contract as well. I also secured signed consent forms to collaborate with the child protection worker and a local police officer involved with their case.

Through the use of the family portrait drawing, the parents in this case were confronted in a powerful way and began to take responsibility for their problematic behaviors. Sandra's drawing successfully reached a place in the parents' minds that served as the impetus for committing to changing their destructive behaviors. Interestingly enough, the parents disclosed in our session that no therapeutic intervention had had more of an "emotional impact" on them than Sandra's family portrait drawing.

Integrating Narrative Therapy Ideas

Michael White and David Epston's Narrative Therapy approach fits theoretically with the Solution-Focused Brief Therapy model in several ways. Both approaches share strong Batesonian influences, are family empowerment models, and capitalize on family members' strengths and resources. The leading proponents of these models believe strongly that children should be advisers on their own lives (de Shazer & White, 1996). However, some important elements of the narrative approach are unique to this model and I have integrated them into the Solution-Focused Brief Therapy model.

Narrative therapists approach cases with a political lens; that is, they bring gender, cultural, and social justice issues into the therapy room. The Narrative Therapy approach tends to be more meaning-based and historical and makes more room for the family's problem story than does the Solution-Focused Brief Therapy approach (Chang & Phillips, 1993; de Shazer & White, 1996; Jenkins, 1994). By taking the time to elicit the family's story about the problem, narrative therapists can learn a great deal about family beliefs and the various ways family members influence and are influenced by the oppressive problem. With this important information, the narrative therapist can engage in externalizing conversations (White, 1995; White & Epston, 1990) with the family to tease out story lines of competency which can help liberate them from their dominant problem-saturated situation. Externalizing the problem (White, 1995; White & Epston, 1990) is an effective therapeutic pathway to pursue with families that do not respond well to the basic Solution-Focused Brief Therapy approach, have been pushed around by the problem for a long time, have experienced multiple treatment failures, and describe the problem as having a life of its own. Often, families that are therapy veterans such as these do not notice times when they are not pushed around by the problem because such events do not fit with their dominant problem-saturated stories. Some therapy veterans may also interpret a Solution-Focused therapist's overemphasis on the positive as not taking their problem story seriously, being sarcastic, and minimizing their plight.

The following case example demonstrates the effectiveness of externalization (White & Epston, 1990) with a 9-year-old African American boy (Jimmy) and his parents, for whom Jimmy's chronic stealing habit of 3 years had become oppressive. I was the fifth therapist the parents had taken Jimmy to see for his stealing problem.

> Jimmy had been stealing money from his parents since he was 6 years of age. According to the father, he also had a long history of using his "slick fingers" to take things from his teachers' desks. Throughout the initial family interview, the father called Jimmy's stealing problem "slick fingers." The mother referred to Jimmy as being a "slick thief," able to find their money hidden in shoe boxes and other inconspicuous places around the house.
>
> The use of the miracle question (de Shazer, 1988), coping, and pessimistic sequence questions (Berg & Miller, 1992) proved to be unproductive in the interviewing process, so I decided to capitalize on the father's externalizing of the problem into "slick fingers." The "slick fingers" construction of the stealing problem was also much more treatable than the parents other explanations, such as: "He must have a character flaw." "We must have spoiled him." and "He is never happy with what he has."
>
> The parents and Jimmy shared their feelings of frustration and hopelessness about never being able to conquer this problem. Jimmy also disclosed that he had "no control" over his stealing problem. By externalizing the problem in our conversation, the parents began to see how they and Jimmy were being victimized by "slick fingers." As a way to help empower the family to win back control of their lives over "slick fingers," I offered them an "honesty test ritual" (Durrant & Coles, 1991; Epston, 1989) to experiment with.
>
> The parents were instructed to leave money laying out in different locations around the house. After securing a signed

consent form from the parents, I contacted Jimmy's teacher to let her know what we were doing to help defeat "slick fingers." The teacher placed previously stolen items on top of her desk for one week to test out Jimmy's ability to stand up to "slick fingers" and not allow it to push him around. I emphasized to the parents, Jimmy, and the teacher the importance of this being a team effort. I also pointed out that stealing habits do not die easily.

One week later, the family came back in good spirits, reporting a perfect week. Jimmy openly admitted that on two occasions he almost succumbed to "slick fingers" 's attempts to brainwash him to steal, but he fought back with useful self-talk. The parents also admitted that they had some moments of distrust with Jimmy, but avoided the temptation to confront him. The teacher had reported to the parents that there were no signs that "slick fingers" had gotten the best of Jimmy in one week's time.

Since the honesty test strategy proved to be so successful, I continued to use it throughout the course of family therapy. I ended up seeing the family four more times. In our final session together, I threw a party for Jimmy and his parents to celebrate their victory over "slick fingers." The teacher joined the festivities as well.

One of the most unique features of White and Epston's narrative approach is the use of an "audience" of friends, relatives, and significant others in the identified child client's life to bear witness to his or her competencies and to pioneer a new direction within the family and in other social contexts. The telling and retelling of the child's new evolving story of competency is empowering and can create possibilities (deShazer & White, 1996; White, 1995).

White and his colleagues have developed several effective therapeutic rituals that can empower families to gain their freedom from the problem's reign over them (Durrant & Coles, 1991; Epston, 1989; White & Epston, 1990). One quite effective ritual with children's behavioral problems is the Habit Control Ritual. Using this therapeutic ritual, family members keep track of their victories over the problem and the problem's victories over them on a daily basis. The therapist can raise dilemmas with family members around their need to be a unified team rather than caving in to having arguments about the best course of action for defeating the problem or continuing to blame the identified child client for their difficulties. I typically instruct families to work out together to be fit to do battle with the tyrannical problem. Once the family has defeated the problem, we can celebrate the change process by giving the family a party, certificates, ribbons, or trophies (Durrant & Coles, 1991; Epston, 1989; White & Epston, 1990). Celebrating change with families in this manner nicely complements the positive-oriented Solution Focused Brief Therapy approach and is an effective way to further amplify "news of a difference" for them.

Contributions from Winnicott and Other Developmental Theorists

In reviewing the Solution-Focused Brief Therapy literature, there is little mention of the importance of developmental theory in informing what we do clinically with children and their families. Having a good grasp of developmental theory can aid us in determining how best to communicate with the child and with designing and selecting therapeutic tasks that he or she is capable of understanding and performing. As Winnicott said: "One must have in one's bones a theory of the emotional development of the child and the relationship of the child to the environmental factors" (1971b, p. 3). For the remainder of this section, I discuss important contributions from Winnicott and other developmental theorists that therapists should consider in their clinical work with children and their families. Winnicott (1971b) always took into account the strengths and resources of the child, as well as the parents' availability and capability to facilitate the child's maturational process. He believed that clients want to be co-collaborators and inevitably guide therapists toward what they really need. When stuck with a case, Winnicott knew how to tolerate and make clinical use of the "not knowing." He had "the capacity to tolerate feeling ignorant or incompetent and a willingness to wait until something genuinely relevant and meaningful emerged" (Casement, 1985, p. 9).

Winnicott (1971b) attempted to create what he called a "holding environment" in which children believe they will get help for their difficulties. He would try to create a natural and free-flowing human relationship, in which clients surprise themselves by sharing important thoughts and feelings (Casement, 1985). Winnicott (1985) believed that some clients' difficulties arise simply because no one has ever "intelligently listened" to their story. Finally, Winnicott practiced somewhat like a brief therapist by increasing the time intervals between sessions once progress occurred.

One of Winnicott's (1971a) most famous play therapy techniques was the Squiggle Game. He would say to the child:

"Let's play something. I know what I would like to play and I'll show you. This game that I like playing has no rules. I just take my pencil and go like that . . . (do squiggle blind). You show me if that looks like anything to you or if you can make it into anything, and afterwards you do the same for me and I will see if I can make something of yours." (pp. 62–63)

Not only does the Squiggle Game help build rapport with the child, but it furnishes the therapist with valuable information about the child's inner world and provides opportunities to indirectly offer children new ideas or solutions to their difficulties. Winnicott believed strongly that therapists working with children had to be able to play and could enjoy playing.

In expanding on Winnicott's Squiggle Game technique, I like to include the parents in the process. I may have the parents draw a squiggle and have the child construct a picture out of the squiggle and tell a story about their picture. The child then draws a squiggle and the parents follow the same procedure. Gil (1994) has also developed another version of the Winnicott Squiggle Game in her clinical work with abused children.

Historically, there has been a heated debate across all mental health disciplines whether "nature" or "nurture" is responsible for childhood problems and personality development. Greenspan (1995) argues that we should instead look at how nature and nurture work in tandem. Using the metaphor of a lock and key to describe the unique and continuous interplay between nature and nurture, Greenspan (1995) says:

> The child brings his "nature" and the parents bring warmth and love wrapped up in a particular pattern of caring. This interplay operates like a lock and key. Finding the right key creates new patterns of interactions. Each stage of child development has its own goals, which are in turn associated with new ways for nature and nurture to work together. For each stage of development, there is a special "key." With the right knowledge about how to find the "keys," parents can learn how to greatly influence this interplay of nature and nurture in their children. (p. 7)

Therapists who treat children need to be knowledgeable about child development. By educating parents on what to expect developmentally with their children and helping them find the right "keys" or course of action for supporting their children's mastery of developmental tasks, we can have a much more meaningful impact on families.

Through the use of education and normalization, therapists can dispel parental concerns about what they and referring persons may be identifying as pathological behaviors. In reality, such behaviors often turn out to be the child's struggle with particular development tasks. As Achenbach (1990) stated:

> Many behavioral/emotional problems for which professional help is sought are not qualitatively different from those most individuals display to some degree at some time in their lives. Instead, many problems for which help is sought are quantitative variations and characteristics that may normally be evident at other developmental periods, in less intense degree, in fewer situations or in ways that do not impair developmental progress. (p. 4)

From a Piagetian cognitive-developmental perspective, Cowan (1978) contends that children's problems, struggles, and conflicts are necessary and inevitable for their growth. At each developmental stage, children have to negotiate optimal personal and environmental mismatches (i.e., the complex interactions between their psychological functioning at a given stage with situational demands and the values of their families, peers, schools, and communities). This can lead to disequilibrations and new problems. In our clinical work with children and their families, we need to encourage parents to be supportive of their child's attempts to cope with these disequilibrations.

For numerous reasons, most family therapists fail to use developmental theory to guide their assessment observations and to design appropriate therapeutic tasks. When training and consulting with family therapists, I frequently hear that one's thinking in developmental terms about a particular family member or the identified child client is "too linear" or "not systemic." It is my contention that the child client is not some innocent victim in his or her family drama but, instead, plays an active part in contributing to family stress and difficulties. The child's role in the family drama can be determined by directly observing family interactions in therapy sessions, as well as graphically depicted in the child's art and play activities. We need to be sensitive to the effects of the child's own adaptation to his or her developmental struggles on other family members and how family members, in turn, respond to the child. For example, if parents provide a great deal of assistance to help their child master toilet training, they may enable the child to achieve competence quickly; however, this attempted parental solution can fail in the long run because the child may lack the self-confidence to use the potty alone. The rewards of independence and confidence go to the child who is allowed to try and fail, struggle, and finally succeed. Finally, we also need to look at how family life-cycle issues affect the child's functioning (Carter & McGoldrick, 1988; Haley, 1986).

Flying Out of Center:
The Art of Therapeutic Improvisation

Jazz critic Robert Levin (1987), in describing the creative and brilliant improvisational abilities of the late saxophonist and reedman Eric Dolphy and other pioneers of the Avant-Garde jazz movement, had the following to say: "The new jazz is about learning to fly, to fly out of the center. . . . To fly means to end the pursuit of the original, the given, the order, to break that circle, and to pursue instead the rediscovery of surprise—which is to say the rediscovery of reality and the vital."

Levin's quote captures the essence of how we as therapists can use ourselves to help liberate the families with which we work from their oppressive, dominant problem-saturated stories. Through the use of humor, absurdity, and surprises in the therapeutic process, we can move our clients out of the center, bring back lost spontaneity and playfulness, and alter fixed beliefs and entrenched family interactive patterns that keep them stuck. Similar to what chaos theorists refer to as *fractals*—that is, unique patterns left behind by unpredictable movements (Briggs, 1992) that occur in nature—I want to inject humor and surprises into each family session to help introduce novel ways for family members to look at their original problem-saturated situations.

To fly out of center and be effective improvisators, we have to feel free to step out of our logical and rational minds and allow our creativity to run wild! When flying out of center with a family, a therapist can tell jokes, exploit and exaggerate a family pattern in a humorous way, share anecdotes and stories, use metaphors, and be as unpredictable as possible. The therapeutic experience with children and their families should be a fun, surprising, and, at times, wacky adventure. Two case examples of flying out of center offer possibilities.

Alison, 6 years old, was brought into therapy for "low self-esteem," "isolating herself from the rest of the family," and for looking "depressed." Alison came to the session with her parents. Her 13- and 16-year-old sisters were involved in school-related sporting events so they did not attend our first family session. No precipitant was identified for Alison's symptoms. Earlier in the session, I felt that I had joined well with the parents but failed to connect with Alison. Alison would not say a word to me, even after I asked the imaginary magic wand question (see Chapter 2, this volume) and tried to engage her in a board game on the floor. It appeared that my approach with Alison was too straightforward, and what I really needed to do was something funny and unpredictable. I decided to fake crying and say in a sad childlike way, "I'm telling my mommy that Alison won't play with me" (I put a sad look on my face). Suddenly, Alison began to smile and laugh at me. She then got on the floor and asked to play a board game together. By the end of the session, Alison opened up about what was making her so sad. Apparently, there had been a major decline in the kind of attention she used to get from her father because of his more recent involvement in coaching her sisters' softball teams. Hearing Alison's concerns proved to be a newsworthy experience for the parents, and the father voiced a desire to try to set aside more individual quality time for Alison.

There are many popular children's stories written both in this country and abroad whose main characters, themes, and story lines parallel our young clients' stories. As another way of engaging a child, improvising, and introducing new angles on the child's story, I share with the child and his or her family a story that seems to fit their situation.

Walter, 8 years old, was brought for therapy shortly after his father, Curtis, had gotten custody of him. Walter and his mother, Michele, had a strained relationship and she no longer wanted custody. Following the parental divorce, it had been decided in court that Walter would go live with Michele. According to Curtis, while Walter lived with his mother, she would "yell at him" a lot, "neglect his needs," and "favor Monica," his 10-year-old sister, who also lived with Michele. It was Curtis's hope that Walter would use counseling to get out all of his "bad feelings" about his "awful experiences" living with Michele. Walter looked sad when I first saw him in the waiting room.

When I greeted the family in the waiting room, I observed that Walter was reading Dr. Seuss's *The Cat in the Hat Comes Back*. Thus, in thinking about the pervasive theme in Walter's story of being an "invisible" child when living with his mother, I decided to share the book *Moomin's Invisible Friend* with Walter and Curtis.

The story in many ways parallels Walter's. Moomin, the main character, and a friend Too Ticky, one day brought home a new friend, Ninny, for Moomin's parents and friends to meet. However, nobody could see Ninny because she was invisible. Ninny was being raised by her nasty aunt who was so horrible to Ninny that Ninny became invisible. Moomin's parents and friends were the nicest people in the Moomin Valley. On a daily basis, Moomin, her parents, and the former's friends would treat Ninny very nicely and compliment her. With almost every act of kindness and compliment, a different part of Ninny's body would begin to appear. After some time had passed, most of Ninny's body could be seen except for her head. The Moomins decided one day to take Ninny to the sea to relax and swim. Moominmamma was standing on the edge of a rock hesitant to jump in, for the water was very cold. Moominpappa decided to push his wife into the water. As he snuck up behind her, Ninny thought this was wrong and bit his tail to stop him. While Moominpappa was screaming in pain, Ninny's head suddenly appeared. Everyone jumped for joy! Finally they could see all of Ninny. Ninny was real happy too because she no longer was invisible. Moomin requested that Ninny never make herself invisible again. Ninny said, "Never! Oh, never!" (Jansson, 1962).

After hearing this story, Curtis vowed that he would not allow his son ever to become invisible while living with him. Walter liked the story a great deal, and said he could identify with Ninny. We used this story as a vehicle for discussing his thoughts and feelings about when he lived with the mother. Over time, Walter's view of himself changed, as well as his pessimistic outlook on the future. Curtis was highly invested in building a nurturing relationship with Walter.

Use of Postmodern Therapy Ideas

According to Fruggeri (1992), therapists who consider themselves to be postmodern practitioners should acknowledge their premises, points of view, and biases with their clients. She argues: "It is through this acknowledgment that they [therapists] can observe their own way of constructing the phenomena they are observing and their relationship to them" (p. 50). Postmodern therapists avoid adopting a privileged expert position with their clients by trying not to present them with some "higher truths" or final explanations about their problem situations. Alternative constructions of the client's problem situation and therapeutic tasks are presented in a tentative way: "I wonder if . . . " "Could it be . . . ?" "This task may be useful as an experiment. . . . " Postmodern therapists recognize that there are a multiplicity of views for any given client problem situation, with all views being constructed (Hoffman, 1990).

Family problems are viewed as being an "ecology of ideas" (Bogdan, 1984). Operating from this postmodern perspective, the main role of the therapist is to facilitate the renegotiation of the meaning system within which "the problem" exists. Thus, the therapist actively enters into dialogue with those individuals who maintain the problem definition and becomes a collaborator in the construction of new client narratives (Anderson & Goolishian, 1988b, 1991a, 1991b). The family can be invited to share with the therapist which involved helping professionals are part of the problem system and with whom the therapist should collaborate.

In a fascinating postmodern study with expert practitioners from a variety of professional disciplines, including therapists, Schon (1983) discovered that these practitioners utilized two processes when managing work tasks: *reflection-in-action* and *reflection-on-action*. He found that the critical reflective thinking that the practitioners employed in their work was an artistic process, not purely a cognitive process of analysis and speculation. For Schon (1983), reflection-in-action is the capacity to keep alive and improvise in the midst of an action that did not require the practitioners to stop and think. Reflection-on-action consists of asking oneself questions about action taken from a critical lens.

In a therapy context, reflection-on-action entails thinking about one's motivations for behaving in a particular way in a session (questions asked and/or interventions tried) and what aspects of the client's story one had taken most seriously (problem-saturated beliefs or solution talk). With reflection-on-action, a therapist seeks new ways of approaching a client's problem situation in a future therapy session, accepts the possibility that the client's problem situation may not fit any pattern of understanding in the therapist's present repertoire, or accepts that he or she has tried to make the client's problem situation conform to a particular theoretical orientation. When we find techniques that are unusually effective with particular client situations, in similar case situations the memory of that response jumps to the forefront of our minds, and we try out the same techniques again to see if they work. If they do, the initial registration or "logging" of their success in our memory is reaffirmed, and the same set of techniques may well become a tried and trusted response to situations characterized by similar patterns. In other words, it becomes a theory in use (Brookfield, 1987; Schon, 1983).

One famous reflective practitioner was the great physicist Niels Bohr. Bohr was never fond of axiomatic systems and declared repeatedly: "Everything I say must be understood not as an affirmation but as a question" (cited in Capra, 1988, p. 18). In a similar vein, psychology researcher and critic Robin M. Dawes argues: "Responsible practitioners should practice with a cautious, open and questioning attitude" (1994, p. 31). Through the use of reflection-in-action and reflection-on-action, we can become better improvisers, be more critical of our therapeutic assumptions and interventions, and be more therapeutically flexible.

OVERVIEW OF THE BOOK

The remainder of the book is designed to provide clinicians with the practical "how-to's" for conducting an integrative Solution-Focused Brief Therapy approach with children and their families. Chapter 2 describes an efficient and comprehensive solution-oriented family assessment method. This family assessment format is structured so that clinicians can gather important child and family background information and establish realistic goals and treatment plans with families in their initial interviews.

Chapter 3 presents five interventive questions that therapists can use to challenge outmoded family beliefs, to elicit family members' strengths, and to get unstuck in the treatment process. The reversal and imagination questions described in this chapter are particularly useful for creating possibilities with children and their families.

Chapters 4 and 5 are both devoted to therapeutic task design and selection. In Chapter 4, I describe how therapists can find *fit*, that is, designing or selecting a therapeutic task that fits with family members' unique cooperative response patterns and problem definitions and the strengths and resources they bring to treatment. Five useful idea-generating strategies for creating novel solutions are also presented. Chapter 5 describes a variety of family play and art therapy tasks that can effectively bring back or promote spontaneity, fun, and other important changes in the child's family. The use of imagination and visualization techniques are also presented in this chapter.

In Chapter 6, I provide practical guidelines for optimizing therapeutic cooperation with families in second and subsequent sessions. I discuss specific strategies and techniques for amplifying and promoting changes with families.

Chapter 7 is devoted to describing effective strategies for collaborating with involved helping professionals from larger systems. I discuss key elements in successful collaborative relationships.

Chapter 8 addresses therapeutic options for getting unstuck with what we would all refer to as "impossible" cases. In this chapter I discuss the use of the identified child client's friend as an expert consultant, the reflecting team, pattern intervention strategies with parents, and the Buddhist stance of nondoing.

Chapter 9 provides practical guidelines for therapists in helping children and their families succeed in a managed care treatment context.

Finally, Chapter 10 summarizes the major themes of the book and offers some implications for future clinical work with children and their families.

CHAPTER 2

The Solution-Oriented Family Assessment Interview: An Efficient and Comprehensive Evaluative Method

When you know what you already don't know you
know, things will happen in even better ways!
                                        –JOHN FRYKMAN

Child psychotherapists and many family therapists have traditionally viewed the diagnostic evaluation or assessment process as a separate stage of therapy that needs to be completed first before the *real* treatment can begin. It is still common clinical practice among child psychotherapists to evaluate and treat the child separately from the parents. Moreover, many therapists maintain the need for a few sessions to arrive at an accurate diagnosis for the child. Some family therapists operating from the "functionalist" school of thought (Bogdan, 1986) may need a session or two to determine the "function of the symptom" (Haley, 1987) and structural family pathology, such as "enmeshment" and "disengagement" (Minuchin, 1974). Yet, in today's managed care world, most therapists only have one assessment session authorized to arrive at a DSM-IV diagnosis and to construct with the client an appropriate treatment plan. Therefore, therapists not only need to learn how to conduct assessment sessions in an efficient manner but also need to be able to negotiate solvable client problems and goals and design realistic treatment plans with children and their families in their first family sessions.

In this chapter, I present a solution-oriented family assessment session format that is not only comprehensive and efficient but designed to create possibilities with clients in their very first family sessions. I discuss key interviewing methods for securing sufficient information regarding the referral process, presenting problems and concerns, child and family developmental and background information, cultural and gender issues, and family members' resiliencies. This discussion is followed by another about how to collaboratively construct treatment plans with families consisting of well-formed client treatment goals and a clear therapeutic action plan. Finally, I conclude the chapter with a discussion on postassessment session critical reflection.

SOLUTION-ORIENTED FAMILY ASSESSMENT SESSION FORMAT

After taking the time to sufficiently connect with each family member about his or her personal strengths and talents, I explain the assessment session format. I share with the family the following description of the format:

> "There are two parts to this assessment session, the first part has to do with talking about the difficulties and concerns that lead to your coming in at this time, and in the second part of the session, we will talk about solutions and change, where you want to be when we have a successful outcome here."

By structuring the assessment session this way, the therapist empowers the family by confidently conveying to them that there are solutions for their difficulties and his or her own belief that the family has the strengths and resources to change. Research supports this stance in that therapists' expectations and beliefs in their clients' abilities to change have been found to have a great deal of influence on treatment outcome (Campbell, 1996; Gingerich, de Shazer, & Weiner-Davis, 1988; Leake & King, 1977; Thomas, Polansky, & Kounin, 1955). Those families that have already experienced multiple treatment failures are pleasantly surprised by encountering a confident, optimistic therapist, ready to discuss their concerns yet also interested in their areas of competency and in rapidly steering them toward change.

This format also allows the clinician to get enough information to complete the forms required by many managed care companies directly following the session. Whenever possible, it's also in the assessor's best interest to call the case manager on the same day of the assessment session to discuss the case and provide a good estimate of the number of visits needed to complete treatment with the clients. Thus, future appointments can be scheduled without delay. With practice, therapists will discover that it is possible to use the first half of the assessment session time to gather a sufficient amount of information about the presenting problems, the child and family background, past treatment experiences, and school functioning to fill out the managed care company's assessment summary forms and, in the same hour-long session, open up the door for change and possibilities for the clients.

The Solution-Oriented family assessment format consists of five major areas of therapeutic inquiry and collaboration:

1. Problem defining and clarification
2. Meaning making: eliciting the family story
3. Assessing the customer(s) for change in the client system
4. Solutions and change: coauthoring a new family story
5. Collaborative treatment planning

To a great degree, all these areas of inquiry and collaboration blend together and complement one another to provide the therapist with a good understanding of the family's problems, beliefs, and goals. For example, when collaborating with families about problem definitions and explanations, we are also engaged in the meaning-making process. However, the meaning-making process goes well beyond problem defining and clarification; it also includes referral process and treatment history, including major illnesses and medications; inquiring about family member's attempted solutions and resiliencies; assessing child and family developmental issues; assessing gender and cultural issues and how they may affect the presenting problems; and assessing who is most motivated to do something about the presenting problems in the client system.

In the second half of the family assessment session, the therapist can inquire with the family about pretreatment changes and solutions to help them begin to coauthor a new problem-free family story. As part of the collaborative treatment planning process, treatment goals are negotiated into solvable terms, treatment modalities and an action plan are agreed upon, and a DSM-IV diagnosis is selected with the family's input. Like the four Buddhist mind-training principles discussed later in this chapter, the self-reflection part of the postassessment session serves as another helpful check to prevent us from becoming too wedded to any one way of thinking about the family, to maintain a curious and open stance, and to be critical of what we chose to do, avoided doing, or forgot to explore or do with the family in a session.

Prior to discussing the five major assessment areas of inquiry, I first discuss four Buddhist mind-training principles that can help therapists in gathering client background information and in listening to clients' problem stories. By listening to our clients with a "beginner's mind," therapists can avoid the common mental trap of trying to understand their clients' problem stories and family situations too quickly.

THE BUDDHIST ASSESSOR WITH A TWIST

When conducting family assessment sessions with children, therapists need to operate from the Buddhist stance of "don't know mind" (Barrett, 1993; Mitchell, 1988), which is forever fresh, open, and fertile with possibilities (Selekman, 1993). The bottom line is that our clients are better experts on their lives than we are. We have to give them plenty of space to share their stories to help us better understand their world views and difficulties. However, research indicates that many therapists have a tendency to formulate their diagnostic impressions within the first 30 to 60 seconds of observing their clients in assessment interviews (Gauron & Dickson, 1969; Yager, 1977). Dawes (1994), in providing an explanation for how therapists arrive so quickly at diagnostic impressions and labels for their clients, argues:

> The heuristics that we use for assessing our clients: *availability* (searching in one's memory for cases similar to the one in front of us) and *representativeness* (matching cues or characteristics with a stereotype or a set of other characteristics associated with a category), most commonly lead to inaccurate case formulations. (p. 130)

The following four Buddhist mind-training principles serve as helpful guidelines for therapists when conducting assessment interviews with children and their families. Therapists will find that all four of the principles can help us to be better listeners and to maintain an open and curious mind when gathering information from family members and trying to understand their client's problem stories.

Pull Out the Rug

There once was a wise teacher in India named Saraha. He often said to his students:

> Those who believe that everything is solid and real are stupid, like cattle, but that those who believe that everything is empty are even more stupid. Everything is changing all of the time, and we keep wanting to pin it down, to fix it. So whenever you come up with a solid conclusion, let the rug be pulled out. (Chodron, 1994, p. 19)

This story captures the essence of the mental traps that therapists tend to fall into when assessing their clients. Chodron (1994) suggests that whenever our thoughts become solid, we should "self-liberate even the antidote" and label our thoughts as "thinking." By doing this, we begin to see the transparency of our thoughts, their illusory nature, and "acknowledge that you just made them all up with this conversation you are having with yourself" (Chodron, 1994, p. 20). We need to let go of small-mindedness and fixation on any particular explanation for the child or family's difficulties by pulling the rug out from under our belief systems.

Cultivate Patience

One therapeutic skill not typically taught in postgraduate family therapy training programs and in workshops is the gentle art of being patient with our clients. We need to learn how to become better observers and listeners. Tao-Wu once said: "If you want to see it, see into it directly; but when you stop to think about it, it is altogether missed" (cited in Barrett, 1993, p. 51). Whenever Erickson would make an observation in a therapy session, he would write it down on a piece of paper, put it in an envelope, and stick it in his desk drawer. Later, he would pull it out and compare it to other observations he had made to see whether there was any consistency to what he was observing with his clients (Erickson & Havens, 1985).

My colleagues and I once had a case in which the mother, a pediatric nurse, was convinced that her 11-year-old son, Bill, was clinically depressed. Bill had been "isolating himself" from the family, appeared to have "low self-esteem," and became "increasingly more noncommunicative." At the intersession break, all three of my colleagues were unanimously convinced that Bill was depressed because he was so "soft spoken," "slouched low" in the corner of the couch, and kept his "head down" for the first half of the session. As the interviewer, I had similar observations. Yet I remained open to the possibility that Bill's nonverbal attitude and soft-spoken voice could indicate any of the following: normative preadolescent behavior, his upset about his parents making him go for counseling (after all he was not even a window shopper for counseling; the parents were the real customers), and the possibility that Bill's demeanor had always been this way. It was not until our second session with this family 4 weeks later that my colleagues began to view Bill differently, particularly when both his parents had very positive reports about his behavioral changes between sessions. Interestingly enough, Bill's nonverbal attitude and soft-spoken voice had not changed at all!

This case helps demonstrate the common therapist mental trap, "What you will see is what you will get." By being patient with my observations and impressions with Bill's case, I left the door open for many possibilities for viewing his situation.

When listening to our clients share their problem stories, we need to try to suspend our own therapeutic agendas, forget about what questions we might want to ask next, and concentrate deeply on the language, themes, and beliefs the clients use to describe their situations. Nichols (1995) contends that "a good listener is a witness, not a filter for your experience" (p. 17). We have to be careful not to allow our personal and therapy model assumptions to determine what we hear from our clients. By listening intently to our clients' descriptions of their problem situations, we can get to know the problem's nature and let it teach us what it will.

Take a Bigger Perspective

There is a sacredness to our clients' wisdom about their problem stories. For them, the map is the territory (Hoffman, 1990). Some families may come to the assessment session armed with a DSM-IV label to which they are wedded and for which they are seeking a confirmation. Rather than trying to talk them out of this DSM-IV label or reframing the problem, therapists need to respect their unique understanding of their problem situations (Selekman, 1996). As therapists, we need to be curious about the second and third possible explanations for a client's presenting problem. The client's response to our questions should be followed up with more curiosity and questions, to enlarge the meaning of their problem story. We will never find the final explanation for the client's story because knowledge is "always on the way." Frank Howell, the famous Native American painter put it best when he said, "We need to create 'windows' which other people can't make for themselves—windows that provide the way to a greater awareness" (cited in Wood & Howell, 1993, p. 7). What prevents our clients from adopting a bigger perspective and creating "windows" for themselves are the emotions and outmoded beliefs that keep them stuck.

Another technique in assessment sessions that can help families adopt a bigger perspective on their problem situations is to ask problem-tracking questions (O'Hanlon & Weiner-Davis, 1989; Palazzoli, Boscolo, Cecchin, & Prata, 1980; Selekman, 1993). Asking a family member to provide a very detailed, videotape-like description of what every family member does when the identified child client is symptomatic or acting up and how the family recursively interacts with one another can help interactionalize the problem and challenge outmoded family beliefs that the genesis and the maintenance of the problem resides in the child being assessed. Problem-tracking questions also help to assess how family members interact with involved helpers representing larger systems, such as school personnel who are concerned about the identified child client. In some cases, the same interactive dance occurring between the parents and the identified child client at home gets played out between the child and his or her teachers and other involved school personnel.

The Tao That Can Be Spoken Is Not the Ultimate Tao

Applied to the world of therapy, the principle "The Tao that can be spoken is not the ultimate Tao" means that when the therapist becomes wedded to one way of looking at the client's presenting problem, he or she cannot see or hear anything else. Our choice therapy models are not a panacea for every client presenting problem situation. Lao-tzu used to teach his students that "the more you know, the less you understand" (Mitchell, 1988, p. 47). As mentioned earlier, by using curiosity and cultivating patience with our clients, we can avoid falling into the tunnel-vision mental trap.

One of my favorite Dr. Seuss short stories, which is a nice metaphor for this Buddhist principle, is the tale of *The Sneetches*. On the beaches there were two types of Sneetches, star-bellied ones and Sneetches without stars. The star-bellied Sneetches held their heads up high and viewed themselves as being superior to the Sneetches without stars on their bellies. The latter were always excluded from the star-bellied Sneetches' hot dog roasts and marshmallow-toasting parties. The plain-bellied Sneetches spent most of their days "moping and doping" on the beaches, until one day a man drove up to them in a strange-looking car. His name was Sylvester McMonkey McBean, who called himself the "Fix-It-Up-Chappie." He pushed some levers and buttons on his car and it turned into a "star-on" machine. For $3 apiece, all the plain-bellied Sneetches went through his machine to get the highly prized stars put on their bellies. The Sneetches were so happy with their star bellies that they rushed over to the original star-bellied Sneetches to show off their beautiful new bellies. The original star-bellied Sneetches were defensive and made it clear to the other Sneetches that they would always be the first star-bellied Sneetches. In the heat of their anger, McBean appeared with another machine which he called a "star-off" machine. For $10 per Sneetch, he convinced the original star-bellied Sneetches that stars were out of style and that having a plain belly was presently "in" and more contemporary. After having their stars removed, they approached the other Sneetches to show off their new look and make it clear to them that they were the superior ones. This greatly angered the original plain-bellied Sneetches who then approached McBean. In a very clever and cunning way, McBean convinced the original plain-bellied Sneetches to have their stars removed. Finally, both groups of Sneetches ended up exhausting all their finances having the stars removed and put back on again and so on. After McBean drove off, now a rich man, both groups of Sneetches decided together that "Sneetches are Sneetches, and no kind of Sneetch is the best on the beaches" (Seuss, 1961, p. 24).

PROBLEM DEFINING AND CLARIFICATION

Most creative problem-solving experts and researchers would argue that problem finding is more important than solution finding (Csikszentmihalyi & Getzels, 1970; Dillon, 1992; Getzels, 1992; Mackworth, 1965; Van Gundy, 1988). Many therapists in this age of managed health care have a tendency to be too solution-minded rather than problem-minded. Finding the "quick" solution becomes our primary goal, when, in fact, achieving a clear understanding of the clients' perceptions of their "real" problems should be our focus in the first half of our family assessment sessions.

Not taking the time to explore with the family what they view as the real problem and editing their problem-saturated story too quickly early in the session inevitably leads to generating solutions unlikely to work in the long run. Therefore, it is critical to take time with our clients to allow curiosity about how they view their problems, why they think their problems exist, which one troubles them the most, and what the consequences of the problem have been. In close collaboration with our clients, we need to discover what problem they feel should be the primary focus of our attention. Problems are not static or fixed but are in a constant state of evolution. The better we clarify with clients the different problem states and further build on our perceptions of their problems, the more likely we will be able to arrive at a problem definition that best captures what the clients view as the "right" problem.

In the problem-finding inquiry with families, asking productive questions about their presenting problems is often more important and a greater achievement than generating any solutions. Van Gundy (1988), a problem-solving expert and researcher, contends that once we have successfully found the right problem in a broader problem situation, "our problem will be resolved." He further adds: "I have termed this product a *problution*, to symbolize the close relationship between problems and solutions" (p. 18). Swedish family therapists Salamon and Grevelius (1996) have found in their innovative clinical work with families that eliciting from the families their "key questions" about their problem situations provides important clues for solution finding. Two examples of key parental questions might be as follows:

"Do you think he has anger inside about the divorce?"

"What should we do as parents [to try to solve the problem]"?

Some examples of productive problem-finding questions are as follows:

"If there was one question that you were dying to ask me about your problem situation, what would that question be?"

"In what ways can I be most helpful to you?"

"What's your theory about why this problem exists?"

"If there was one question that you were hoping I would ask you while we are working together, what would that question be?"

MEANING MAKING: ELICITING THE FAMILY STORY

Therapists never approach a new family with a tabula rasa. Based on the referral information and past experiences, treating similar types of family problems inevitably triggers in the therapist preconceptions about what to explore or observe in the first family interview. Thus, the meaning-making process begins with the referral context. With the referral process, the therapist needs to explore the history of how the family came to pursue therapy (Andersen, 1991). It is helpful to invite family members to share their thoughts about how they ended up at the office by asking them the following questions:

"Who was the first person who got the idea that you should seek help?"

"What idea do you think [referral person from larger system] had that made him or her decide that you need counseling now?"

"Who else thought counseling would be helpful now?"

"Whom did he or she consult with first?"

"How long did it take from the time you had the idea to seek counseling to pursue it?"

"Do you have any idea about what [referral person from larger system] needs to see happen in counseling that would convince him or her that you wouldn't have to come here anymore?"

By securing detailed information about the history of the idea of pursuing therapy, we can learn a great deal about family members' beliefs, who is the most or least concerned about problems, and what helping professionals from larger systems we will need to collaborate with. If there is some discrepancy between what the family tells me about the referral process or their presenting problems and the information I have on my intake form, I explore with the family how they think the intake worker got his or her ideas about their situation and whether there is something else important that we have not yet talked about. Finally, we need to be sensitive to the constraints of the referral treatment context in terms of what can realistically be treated, time factors, and clinic or agency treatment philosophy, policy, and procedures that can influence our therapeutic work with families.

The late family therapy pioneer Harry Goolishian once said, "I learned to listen, understand and converse in the language of my clients, as opposed to the language of my theory" (1990, p. 179). What made Goolishian a masterful meaning maker and storyteller was his uncanny ability to balance listening, curiosity, and the use of the client's language in the therapeutic conversation. Goolishian would "move with the family as they present themselves, with total respect for their rightness" (Phillips, 1986, p. 6). Like Goolishian, when eliciting the family's problem story, we need to listen carefully to the words they use to describe it, their beliefs, and important themes in their stories. We need to avoid being narrative editors and instead serve as consulting coauthors speaking the client's language and being curious about family members' understanding of their family drama, how it has evolved, and where it is going. Through this meaning-making process, shared understandings can develop that did not exist before the family assessment interview.

What is important is that there are multiple meanings to the words that family members use to describe their problem situation and that their problem stories are stories about stories. As Wittgenstein (1963) has pointed out: "Words are not maps of reality. The significance of our words remains open, vague, ambiguous, until they are used in different particular ways in different particular circumstances" (p. 154). For example, the word "run" has 142 different meanings depending on how it is used (Erickson & Havens, 1985, p. 14). Thus, it is important to have family members clarify the meaning of the words they use with others in the therapy room or when describing their problem situation. The whole therapeutic enterprise is an ambiguous process. We may think we really understand a family's situation and are being helpful to the family when, in reality, they believe we are missing the boat. Sometimes the reverse is true as well. "Real understanding of families is but an illusion or delusion that we carry with us" in our clinical work (Newfield, Kuehl, Joanning, & Quinn, 1991, p. 306).

Children's Memory Processes and Meaning Making

Cognitive research with children has found distinct differences between the memory processes of younger and older children and adults. Younger children are less able to direct their memories for the purposes of either storing or retrieving information, and they are less able to monitor the accuracy of their memories than are older children and adults (Gabarino & Stott, 1992). Because young children lack the capacity for metamemory, they know less about their own memories, are less aware of what they remember and do not remember, and are not aware of the possibility of post-event suggestion influencing what they remember (Ceci, Ross, & Toglia, 1987; Saywitz, 1987). When asked to remember past events, younger children are more likely to make errors of omission than are older children and adults (Gabarino & Stott, 1992). It is not until they are 11 or 12 years of age that children's deliberate recall abilities are as well developed as adults' (Cole &

Loftus, 1987; Gabarino & Stott, 1992). Younger children in particular need contextual support to retrieve their memories—that is, any experiences, people, or objects from the context in which a memory was originally encoded (Daehler & Greco, 1985).

In summarizing the clinical implications of the previous cognitive research studies, therapists need to keep in mind four important findings when assessing and interviewing children:

1. The age of the child determines his or her cognitive capacity to retrieve, identify, and interpret the content of his or her memories.

2. Younger children's capacity to retrieve memories can be enhanced through the use of contextual support (Daehler & Greco, 1985), such as using human figurines and puppets, dollhouses, and art supplies to help them express their interpretations of their family stories.

3. Children are highly susceptible to the postevent suggestions and ideas offered by parents, teachers, significant others, and therapists; subsequently, when listening to children's stories about critical events in their lives, we may be hearing children echoing someone else's voice or interpretation.

4. When remembering postevents, young children are more likely to make errors of omission; therefore, therapists need to be careful not to accept children's stories as complete and accurate accounts of reality.

Assessing Family Members' Attempted Solutions

As an integral part of the meaning-making process, therapists need to explore in great detail with the family what their attempted solutions have been and what their resiliencies (successful individual and family coping and problem-solving strategies) are. It is most helpful to explore with the parents everything they have tried to do on their own to resolve their child's difficulties. I like to ask parents some of the following questions when inquiring about their attempted solutions:

"Has anything you tried in the past to resolve other difficulties with your child worked that we might want to test out with this new problem?"

"Has there been anything that you thought about trying, maybe something off the wall, but you held back because you didn't think it would work?"

"When your son misbehaves, what do the two of you typically do to manage his behavior?"

The answers can furnish the therapist with important information regarding areas for parental intervention and potential building blocks for solution construction. It is also important to find out from identified child clients what their attempted solutions have been when they were pushed around by the problem.

Another area to explore with families that have been in treatment before is what they liked and disliked about former therapists. I like to empower families by placing them in the expert position in designing the kind of treatment experience they would like to have with me. Such questions as the following can be asked:

"You have seen a lot of therapists before me; what did they miss with your situation?"

"What kinds of things should a counselor do with a family like yours?"

"If you could describe what the perfect counselor would be like for you and your family, what would he or she be like?"

"If I were to work with another family just like yours, what advice would you give me to help that family out?"

For families that have not had treatment before, I like to plant the idea that they are more ripe for change than families that have had lots of previous treatment.

Assessing Family Members' Resiliencies

The therapist should also inquire about family members' and family group resiliencies. I share with families that I am very interested in their strengths, particularly in learning about the various ways as individuals and as a group that they have successfully managed past and present stressful life events. I ask the following questions:

"Can you think of any past life events or crisis situations that were pushing your family around, and yet you weathered the storm?"

"What did you do as a family to pull that off?"

"What else did you do as a family that seemed to help?"

"Mom and Dad, can you think of a time in the past when your child was struggling to cope with a painful life event/transition? What did you do to help him or her better cope and get back on track?"

(*To parents*) "Have you noticed anything your daughter does that seems to help her be less stressed out?"

"Can you think of anything that your mom and dad could do to help you better deal with your grandpa's death?"

"What do you do that seems to work in helping you deal with your parents splitting up?"

"When you were your son's age, what did you do to bounce back when you were teased and bullied at school?"

The answers to these questions can provide the therapist with a wealth of information about key family member and family group resiliencies which can be harnessed and channeled into the presenting problem area. It has been my clinical experience that family members take pride and joy in sharing past triumphs in successfully managing a painful or stressful life event.

Assessing Child and Family Developmental Issues

When inquiring with parents about their child's developmental issues, past illnesses, prescribed medications, and psychosocial functioning, it is important to remember that the child developmental theories we use as frameworks for assessing the child are not carved in stone. Each child we interview is unique and does not typically experience a smooth transition from one developmental stage to the next. Observed behavior may not account fully for the child's underlying capacities. It is also important when assessing a child's development to be critical of our conclusions and try to consider how things might look and feel to the child. Besides asking parents about their child's mastery of major developmental milestones, I like to gather information about the child's functioning in the following seven areas: self-awareness, mood management, problem-solving capacity, self-motivation, empathy for others, social competence, and school functioning. When exploring with the parents about their child's functioning in these areas, it is important to find out how well the parents are coping with their child's developmental struggles, particularly how they typically respond to the child. Where the child is at developmentally dictates the level of skill development in each of these areas. I look for certain things in each of the skill areas and I ask parents certain kinds of questions when gathering information about the child's mastery level in these areas.

Self-Awareness

The child appears to know what he or she is feeling. He or she is congruent with his or her thoughts and feelings. When upset, the child can readily express him or herself to the parents. The child displays a good understanding of changes that occur around him or her in the home environment and in other social contexts.

Questions: When your child is sad/mad/happy can she express herself? Does he appear to be aware of his feelings when he looks sad or angry? Can your daughter express to you when she is having difficulties coping with changes/stressors/crises at home? Does his words seem to match how he looks when expressing himself?

Mood Management

This is the child's capacity to self-soothe when anxious, feeling bad, or under a great deal of stress. The child also has the capacity to bounce back quickly from setbacks.

Questions: Does your child appear to have the ability to comfort herself when upset (sad/mad)? How well does your child manage disappointments? How long does it typically take for your child to rebound from feeling frustrated/sad/angry? Does he rebound quickly or slowly? Do your child's moods fluctuate a lot or are they pretty balanced? What does your son typically do when he is frustrated/mad/sad?

Problem-Solving Capacities

The child is skilled at managing tasks through completion. He or she has no difficulty staying focused and concentrating on the task at hand. The child acts rather than reacts to daily and life challenges.

Questions: When faced with a challenging or upsetting situation, what does your son typically do? Does he tend to think things through before taking action or does he react impulsively? When you and your daughter are at odds, how does she typically respond?

Self-Motivation

The child approaches tasks and challenges with desire and enthusiasm. Parents and other significant adults do not have to be the motivating force for the child. The child takes responsibility for completing assigned tasks, such as chores or putting toys away when done playing with them.

Questions: Does your child take the initiative to get chores/homework done or do you have to be the motivating force to get the job done? When involved with a new sports activity or task, does he commit to it through completion or does he lose interest quickly and want to give up?

Capacity for Empathy

Although children by nature show signs of empathy for others before becoming toddlers, the capacity for adultlike empathy does not occur until they are 5 to 7 years of age (Greenspan, 1995). At this time, they can begin to see the world through the others' eyes and try to comfort others in distress.

Questions: Does your child show concern for or try and provide support for others when they are in distress? Is your child sensitive to your needs and expectations? And to her brothers' and sisters' needs and feelings?

Social Competence

Between the ages of 7 and 8, the child seeks peer group affiliation (Greenspan, 1995). The child has to master the ability to negotiate multiple relationships, learn how to assess group dynamics, and perform well in group activities. The child has the ability to make and sustain friendships.

Questions: Does your child have any difficulties making and sustaining friendships? Does your child have a close friend? In group situations, does your child tend to withdraw or socialize freely with confidence?

School Functioning

The child has no difficulties with auditory and visual memory or perceptual processes, with staying on task, and with completing assignments and tasks. He or she is able to follow directions and respect the classroom rules and the teacher's authority; he or she has no behavioral problems or difficulties with other students. The child displays the ability to delay gratification, ask for help when necessary, and express opinions or needs.

Questions: Does your child have any difficulties academically or with the learning process? Has the teacher voiced any concerns with your son's ability to stay on task, complete assignments, or get along with peers in the classroom? Are there any reported problems with following the rules or testing the teacher's limits? Any problems with doing, completing, or turning in homework assignments?

By gathering this important developmental information from the parents and the child, we can collaboratively identify target areas for intervention, elicit valuable information about the child's strengths and competency areas, negotiate treatment goals, and have the family assist us with therapeutic task selection and construction.

Family developmental life-cycle issues are also important to consider as part of the meaning-making process. For example, symptoms may develop in a child going to school for the first time or following the birth of the second child in the family. One way to look at the firstborn child's symptomatic behavior is as a normative protest to being dethroned by the newborn. He or she will now have to share center stage in the family, which is a major adjustment for most children.

Gender and Cultural Issues

Two final areas to assess in the meaning-making process are gender and cultural issues. It is helpful to assess in what ways power imbalances among family members and patriarchal assumptions contribute to the maintenance of the presenting problems. Recently, I treated a family in which the 6-year-old identified child client was "depressed" and "diagnosed by the school as exhibiting ADD." In the family assessment session, the mother proceeded to blame herself for her son's problems and cited a multitude of reasons why her husband could not participate in family therapy. At the same time, she disclosed how she felt "all alone" with her son's "problems" and wished she could "go out with girlfriends more." I gently challenged the mother's patriarchal-based beliefs that it was up to her to resolve her son's problems alone and that she should sacrifice her social life for the sake of motherhood. In reflecting on her own mother, she disclosed how her mother too was oppressed by traditional values and expectations about how women should be. We agreed that it was necessary for her husband to participate in future family therapy sessions and that she should have a life outside the family. She confronted her husband a few hours after our session about the need for him to come to the next appointment. She also made plans with some longtime friends to go away for a weekend. The husband's involvement in subsequent family therapy sessions helped us to quickly resolve their son's difficulties; probably because the son had reported that his father's absence from the home, due to several business trips, was why he was feeling "sad" and having problems in school.

Feminist family therapists have argued that most family therapy and brief therapy models fail to address power imbalances between family members, do not challenge traditional patriarchal assumptions about women's role behaviors, and view the importance of establishing a nonhierarchal therapeutic relationship with women and their families (Bograd, 1990; Goodrich, 1991; Luepnitz, 1988; Walsh & Scheinkman, 1989; Whipple, 1996). In discussing the myth of therapeutic neutrality, Avis (1986) contends that "therapists who adhere to this myth inadvertently adopt political positions by what they choose to focus on, respond to, challenge, or ignore, which may reinforce traditional values oppressive to women" (p. 217).

The last important assessment area to explore in the meaning-making process with families is cultural issues that are interwoven with their problem stories and played out in the context of the therapeutic relationship. When working with families from different ethnic and cultural backgrounds, we need to ask ourselves the following questions:

[If you are a white therapist] "Have I examined my own white identity in terms of what it means to be white in our society?"

"How do I feel about being white and my own ethnic and/or cultural background?"

"How does being white and/or being from a different ethnic or cultural background affect what I can see, hear, and think about this family?"

"In what ways does being white in our society grant me with privileged status?"

"How does this privileged status and power imbalance affect my relationships with the African American families I am working with?"

"If you were African American, Asian, Latino, how comfortable would you feel working with a white therapist?"

"What would your concerns be with a white therapist?"

According to Pinderhughes (1990), therapists must learn how to monitor and manage "feelings, perceptions and attitudes mobilized as a result of one's clinical and cultural group status role" (p. 133) in order to have effective culturally sensitive clinical practices. Therapists should utilize curiosity as a respectful way to try to better understand the client's cultural background.

Other important areas to explore with families from different ethnic and cultural backgrounds are the various ways they are oppressed and marginalized by particular groups in our society, negative discriminatory interactions with larger systems representatives, how they feel about working with a therapist of another ethnic and/or cultural background, and whether or not they would like a referral to a therapist with the same ethnic and/or cultural background. Finally, with families that are new immigrants, it is important to assess how well the family members are adjusting to such transitional stressors as language barriers and dramatic differences in religion, education, family values, and lifestyles (Landau-Stanton, 1990; Sluzki, 1979). When there is transitional conflict occurring with immigrant families, we may observe such difficulties as social isolation, extremes in family boundaries, either being too loose or too rigid, and parent–child conflicts related to cultural disharmony, such as the child's attempts to break ties with traditional family values and adopt mainstream societal values (Landau-Stanton, 1990).

ASSESSING THE CUSTOMER(S) FOR CHANGE IN THE CLIENT SYSTEM

De Shazer (1988) has developed a highly practical and useful therapeutic guide for determining who in the client system is most motivated to work with the therapist in resolving the presenting problem. In some cases, the real customers for change may be the referring person or other involved helping professionals from larger systems. De Shazer (1988) has identified the following three different therapist–family relationship patterns: visitors, complainants, and customers. These therapist–family relationship patterns are not fixed but change as the therapist develops *fit* (de Shazer, 1985) and cooperative working relationships with family members. It is important to remember that each family member has a unique cooperative response pattern and may be at a different stage of change (Prochaska, Norcross, & DiClemente, 1994). Therefore, therapists needs to match their questions and therapeutic tasks carefully with the stage of change and unique cooperative response patterns of each family member.

Descriptions of the three different types of therapist–family relationship patterns are followed here by case illustrations highlighting useful therapeutic intervention strategies for each clinical situation.

Visitors

Most children brought for therapy are visitors. It is typically their parents or an outside social control agent who is most concerned about their behavior. When asked about the particular behaviors that parents or the referring person is most concerned about, the visiting child often shrugs his or her shoulders and says, "I don't know," or doesn't respond at all. Older, latency-age children may deny that they have a problem or blame their parents, teachers, or other external factors for their difficulties. Prochaska et al. (1994) contend that visitors are in the "precontemplation" stage of the change cycle. Precontemplators/visitors want their parents and social control agents "off their backs."

In some cases, the whole family could be considered visitors. I like to refer to these families as "no-problem problem" families (Eastwood, Sweeney, & Piercy, 1987) in that not even the parents are alarmed that their child got into trouble at school or in the community. With no-problem problem families, the identified child client is typically a "good student," has never had any major behavioral problems warranting the need for treatment in the past, and is described by the parents as being basically "a good kid."

When working with visitors, we need to be warm and caring hosts and hostesses. We can empathize with the visiting child or parents' dilemma about having to see us for court-ordered or school-referred family therapy and accept whatever goal they may have for themselves. Some children may want help with dealing with their annoying siblings, a problematic peer, one of the parents, or teachers who are always on their back. With a highly oppositional child, it can be helpful to set up a split so that together the therapist and the child can prove the pessimistic referring person wrong: for example, the therapist can have the child pretend to engage in positive prosocial behavior as an experiment in a class in which the child was having difficulties, to "blow the teacher's mind!"

The Columbo approach (see Selekman, 1993, 1995a) is particularly useful when a child or parent is making the therapist feel highly incompetent as a therapist. The television detective Columbo is a master at strategically using his bungling and confused presentational style to throw potential murder suspects off balance and inevitably to lead him to important clues for solving the crime. Similarly, by showing our feelings of incompetence and confusion, the child and the parents will want to be more helpful to us, will be more inclined to clarify the referral process and presenting concerns, and possibly will be more receptive to exploring problem-solving strategies.

If the previous therapeutic strategies fail to foster a cooperative therapist–family relationship or produce a treatment goal, I simply compliment family members on whatever they report doing for themselves that has been good for them, such as showing up for our first scheduled appointment, and I do not offer them therapeutic tasks. The following case example illustrates the utility of the Columbo approach with a no-problem problem family.

> Melissa, a precocious 8-year-old, was school-referred by her teacher because of her "aggressive behavior" in the classroom. This was the third time Melissa had been reprimanded for "kicking and punching" the same male student in her class. The teacher also requested that the school social worker evaluate Melissa for her "violent tendencies." According to Jane, the mother, she was surprised to receive phone calls from both the teacher and the school social worker, for Melissa was an A student and "not violent or aggressive at home." Although Melissa was quite talkative in the session, she denied any family problems or worries early in our session. When asked if she would have ever considered taking Melissa for counseling if the school crisis situation had not occurred, Jane responded with, "Why ... there were no problems." Feeling stuck, I decided to put on my imaginary wrinkled trenchcoat and utilize the Columbo approach.
>
> THERAPIST: (*looking puzzled*) I'm really confused ... help me out with this. Both the teacher and school social worker called you about Melissa's punching and kicking this boy in the class. Do we know if he might have pushed her buttons or was bothering her in some way?

MOTHER: Well . . . I don't know. (*looking at Melissa*) Was that boy annoying you?

MELISSA: Yeah! Jason is always calling me names and bothering me. So I punched him and he kept up so I kicked him. He never quits, I mean I tell him to stop, but he keeps it up.

THERAPIST: How long has he been bothering you?

MELISSA: Since the beginning of the school year.

JANE: You're kidding! Why didn't you tell me, sweetheart?

THERAPIST: Where is the teacher when Jason is pushing your buttons? Do you ever ask for her help?

MELISSA: She doesn't do anything. I mean sometimes she will talk to him, but it doesn't do any good. It felt good to punch him!

THERAPIST: Sounds like you are frustrated and mad about the Jason situation. So if Jason has been bothering you since September, what has stopped you from asking your mother for help with this?

MELISSA: Well, since Miss Brown [the teacher] can't do anything about it . . . what could my mom do?

THERAPIST: (*turning to mother*) I wonder how your daughter got the idea that she could not call upon you for support when the going gets rough for her?

JANE: I don't know . . . I mean I have always been there for her in the past. I have been pretty stressed out a lot lately because of some changes at my job and my husband has been out of town on business quite a bit. (*looking at Melissa*) I'm surprised that you didn't come to me for help way back in September . . . I would have tried to meet with your teacher.

THERAPIST: (*looking at mother*) Do you have any idea what the teacher and school social worker need to see happen in counseling that would convince them that you wouldn't have to come here anymore?

JANE: Well, I guess Melissa would not be punching and kicking Jason or any other students for that matter. (*turning to Melissa*) What do you think, Melissa?

MELISSA: It's going to be hard, Mommy. Jason never quits . . . I mean . . . I will try.

THERAPIST: What do you guys think about the idea of my setting up a meeting at school for the three of us with Miss Brown and the social worker to see if we can together resolve the difficulties between Melissa and Jason?

JANE: That sounds like a great idea! What do you think, Melissa?

MELISSA: Yeah, that sounds fine if it works.

I ended up seeing the family twice in my office and twice in collaborative meetings at the school with the teacher and social worker. In therapy sessions, Melissa and her mother came up with several good ideas for avoiding the temptation to swear at, kick, or punch Jason. In the school meetings, the teacher agreed to refocus her attention on Jason's behavior, which led her to discover that he was instigating fights daily and causing problems with other students. By the time of our first school meeting, the teacher began to notice that Melissa was displaying "good self-control" and "no aggressive behavior."

Complainants

Complainants can be parents, school personnel, or other social control agents. They are typically very concerned or worried about a child's behaviors and want the "expert" therapist to "fix" the child. Often complainants do not include themselves initially when describing the family problem-maintaining interaction patterns, nor do they view themselves as co-collaborators in the solution-construction process. Prochaska et al. (1994) would argue that the complainant is in the "contemplative stage" of the change cycle: He or she recognizes that there is a problem but is not yet ready to take action. Many complainants expect therapists to see their children alone and "figure out why" they "act out" and have "low self-esteem" or "attitude" problems. These parents often claim that their hectic work schedules prevent them from being able to attend their children's therapy sessions regularly.

Because complainants are excellent supersleuths by nature, it makes a great deal of sense for therapists to capitalize on their excellent observational skills by giving them an observation task (de Shazer, 1988; Selekman, 1993). The parent is given the following directive:

> "I am struck by your tremendous insight into your child's behavior, but in order to give me a more complete picture of what we are looking at, I would like you to do a little experiment for me over the next week. I would like you to pull out your imaginary magni-

fying glass and notice all of the encouraging steps [child's name] will be taking on a daily basis. Please write those encouraging steps down and bring that information to our next appointment."

The following case example demonstrates how to engage a complainant who has been involved in multiple treatment experiences for her own alcoholism, as well as for her son's stealing, lying, and ADD. At the beginning of the first interview, I considered William a visitor due to his lack of desire to be in another counseling situation again.

William, a 10-year-old boy, was school-referred for counseling due to his "disruptive, clowning behavior" in the class. His grades were slipping because he failed to complete homework assignments or to turn them in when he did complete them. He also had a tendency to "mouth off" to his teacher when she reprimanded him. On the homefront, Renee, the mother, described William as "always getting under her skin" by "stealing money" from her and "bullying his two younger sisters." According to Renee, William had been stealing from her "since he was a toddler." She also reported that whenever William came back from a weekend visitation with his father, George, he was "totally wired" and "difficult to manage." Renee's two final complaints concerned William's lack of closeness with his stepfather, Steve, and his worsening "ADD condition," despite the fact that his pediatrician had placed him on Ritalin. After getting absolutely nowhere with the miracle question (de Shazer, 1988; see also below), I shifted gears and asked Renee how she managed to cope with all the problems to better cooperate with her pessimism. I decided to meet alone with Renee.

THERAPIST: I am curious how have you managed to cope with all of these difficulties. I mean, some parents would have thrown in the towel already.

RENEE: Well . . . as much as William is a pain in the butt sometimes, I still love him. Who knows . . . maybe it is a self-esteem problem.

THERAPIST: What steps have you taken to prevent this situation from getting worse?

RENEE: Well, I am in regular contact with his teacher and counselor at school. I mean I keep taking him for counseling . . . but it doesn't seem to work. Part of the problem is his father,

George. He is also in recovery, but from drugs. We really can't stand one another. I mean I think he sabotages what Steve and I try and do at home with William.

THERAPIST: With all of your past counseling experiences with William, do you remember if any of the therapists incorporated George into the treatment process?

RENEE: No. None of them did.

THERAPIST: Do you think that could be helpful for me to try and engage his father to work with us to help William?

RENEE: Good luck. He is one of most hard-headed men I have ever met . . . but I guess it is worth a shot.

THERAPIST: Do you think it would also be a good idea for me to collaborate with William's teacher, school counselor, and the pediatrician?

RENEE: Definitely, The school people are totally fed up with William and have discussed the possibility of putting him in a therapeutic day school. I would really like to avoid that at all costs.

By shifting gears and better matching my questions with Renee's pessimistic stance, we did a complete U-turn from my fielding complaints to eliciting her strong desire to help William out and explore potential avenues for solution construction. I also gave Renee an observational task of keeping track, on a daily basis, of the various things she was doing to prevent William's behavior from getting worse, particularly those strategies that seemed to work in eliciting positive responses from him.

In future sessions, I successfully engaged the father around the school's threat of placing William in a therapeutic day school, an outcome he wanted to avoid as well. I was also able to unify the adults around the importance of parental consistency with limit setting and working together as a team when William would try to split them. The teacher and school counselor were very cooperative and I was successful in building a bridge between the school and the home around problem-solving efforts. William's stealing behavior stopped once he was more receptive to learning positive ways to "steal his mother's attention." In collaboration with the pediatrician, we mutually agreed to revisit the Ritalin issue. It turned out that an adjustment in the Ritalin dosage was necessary, and the adjustment helped William to be less hyper and more focused with his school assignments. I ended up seeing the family for 10 sessions over 1 year's time.

Customers

The customer is a parent, the referring person, or another involved helping professional from a larger system who is most concerned about the identified child's problematic behaviors and wants to work closely with the therapist in generating solutions. Ideally, having at least one customer in the family sessions is all it takes to resolve the presenting problem. The same is true at school. If the teacher is the customer, getting him or her to look at the child's behavior differently, abandon unsuccessful attempted solutions, and try new behaviors in response to the child's problematic behaviors can promote changes with the child. The following questions are useful in sessions when the therapist is trying to determine the customer(s) in the client system:

"Who in your family is most concerned about this problem?"

"Who else?"

(*Asking the identified client*) "On a scale of 1 to 10, 10 being most concerned about you, what number would you give everybody in your family?"

"What difference will it make to each person in the family when the problem is solved?"

"If things get worse with this problem situation, who will suffer the most?"

"Who next?"

"Who at school is most concerned about this problem situation?"

"Who else?"

SOLUTIONS AND CHANGE: COAUTHORING A NEW FAMILY STORY

Once the therapist has gathered sufficient family and child background information and clarified with the family what they view as the main problem they want to work on changing first, the second half of the family assessment session is devoted to eliciting from each family member what his or her initial treatment goals and desired outcome pictures will look like. By moving the interview discussion in this positive direction, we are helping the family coauthor a more preferred solution-determined story in which they are the lead authors. As a lead-in to this discussion, I share with the family the following: "Now we can talk about solutions and change—where you want to be when we have a successful outcome here." Sometimes the family and I go into a completely different room when beginning this part of the family assessment session so that we can turn the light switch off on "problem talk" (Gingerich et al., 1988), thus heightening the family's awareness and expectation that something positive and surprising is about to happen. There are four parts to this portion of the family assessment session: goal setting, collaborative treatment planning, the editorial reflection, and postassessment session self-reflection.

Goal Setting

To begin the goal-setting process with the family, I may utilize the miracle question (de Shazer, 1988; de Shazer & White, 1996; Miller & Berg, 1995; Selekman, 1993) or other presuppositional questions (O'Hanlon & Weiner-Davis, 1989; Selekman, 1993) to elicit from each family member what an ideal treatment outcome picture will look like when all their problems are solved. With both of these categories of questions, it is most advantageous to expand the possibilities with each family member—that is, have them spell out in great detail the changes they envision in all their familial and extrafamilial relationships, and in every social context with which they interface, such as the peer group and the school. Family members absent from the assessment session can be introduced into the miracle question inquiry as well, for example, by asking the identified child client the following: "If your father were sitting here, what would he be the most surprised with that changed about you after the miracle happened?"

Miracle Question

When asking the miracle question, it is important that the therapist be patient and give family members plenty of time to think and respond. If they appear to be having difficulty answering the question, I ask them to pretend or play around with the idea that all their problems are magically solved. Typically, this helps open up the imagination doors for family members who are initially having difficulties with the miracle question. The therapist should avoid asking leading questions and allow family members to introduce their own unique solutions and envisioned changes in the miracle picture spontaneously. Once family members have shared their miracle pictures, the therapist can utilize curiosity to explore with them other changes they wondered about that might be happening and to ask whether any of their miracles are happening a little bit already. The miracle question sequence is as follows:

> "Suppose you go home tonight and you go to bed, and while you are sound asleep a miracle happens and all of your problems are solved. When you wake up the next day, how will each of you be able to tell that this miracle really happened?"
>
> "What will be different?"
>
> "What else will have changed with your situation?"
>
> "What difference will that make?"
>
> "What else will be better?"
>
> "Who will be the most surprised—your [mother, father, brother, sister]—when you do that?"
>
> "What effect will that have on your relationship with your mother when you do that more often?"
>
> "How will your mom and dad have changed?"
>
> "When they are yelling less, how will the three of you be getting along better?"
>
> "What else will you be doing instead with your parents?"
>
> "When he does that, how will you [the parents] be treating him differently?"
>
> "How will you get that to happen?"
>
> "What about at school? What will your teacher notice first that changed with you?"
>
> "What else will you be doing instead in class that will help you and your teacher get along better?"
>
> "I'm curious, have there been any times lately when you have seen pieces of this miracle happening already?"
>
> "When was the most recent piece of the miracle?"

With younger children who are cognitively unable to grasp the concept of a miracle, I may hand the identified child client an imaginary magic wand and have him or her wave it in the air and "zap" each family member with it, as well as explore what changes they would make happen with their teacher, friends, or any peers with whom they are having trouble at school or in the neighborhood. After the identified child client is finished, I hand the imaginary magic wand to the parents and siblings present in the family assessment session.

The following case example demonstrates the usefulness of the imaginary magic wand with a 6-year-old boy named Charlie and his parents.

> Charlie was brought for counseling because of his severe temper tantrums and for not responding to his mother's limit setting, particularly when his father was not around.
>
> THERAPIST: If I gave you [Charlie] an imaginary magic wand, careful don't drop it (*reaching over to hand Charlie the wand*), and asked you to wave it in the air to warm it up first and then zap your family with it, how would you make your family better? What would you change first?
>
> CHARLIE: They would be happy . . .
>
> THERAPIST: What would make everyone happy?
>
> CHARLIE: We will play together a lot. Dad will be home more . . .
>
> THERAPIST: What will you play together?
>
> CHARLIE: We don't make puzzles no more . . . I like to make puzzles with Daddy . . . but he's at work a lot.
>
> THERAPIST: When Dad's home more will you make puzzles again?
>
> CHARLIE: Yeah! Daddy . . . Daddy . . . I want to make the airplane puzzle . . . can we?!
>
> MARILYN [mother]: I wonder if this is why Charlie is so upset these days because he misses not playing with you (*looking at George, her husband*)? Matthew [therapist], do you think this is why he is having such bad temper tantrums because he is angry about this?
>
> THERAPIST: I don't know. What do you think about this, George?
>
> GEORGE: Marilyn might be right. I've had to be out of town a lot on business and I can understand why Charlie is so upset. We used to play a lot together in the past. Charlie, what do you think . . . have you been mad because I've been away a lot?
>
> CHARLIE: (*hugging his father*) I miss you . . . I want to play more with you. Can we make the airplane puzzle when we get home?

MARILYN: I miss Daddy too, honey (*looking at Charlie*).

THERAPIST: (*looking at George*) Will your business trip situation be changing soon or will this be a regular part of your job responsibilities?

GEORGE: Yeah, it should be slowing down in a few weeks for awhile. (*looking at Marilyn and Charlie*) I miss you guys a lot when I'm away.

THERAPIST: Charlie, you did a nice job with the magic wand. Are there any other wishes you would like to make come true with it or should we let Mom and Dad have a try with it?

CHARLIE: Here, Daddy (*handing the wand to his father*), you try! What do you wish?

GEORGE: Not as many business trips. Charlie is happy and not mad anymore. We go on a nice family trip together.

THERAPIST: Where do you want to take your family?

GEORGE: Out west . . . maybe the Rockies or the Grand Canyon.

MARILYN: That sounds great. When are we going?

The remainder of the interview was upbeat. When it was Marilyn's turn to use the magic wand, she wished for Charlie to be "happier" and for her husband to be "around more," and she also thought it was "time for a family trip." Earlier in the family assessment session, Marilyn thought Charlie's "temper tantrum" problem was related to his having "low self-esteem," "looking depressed," and having "anger management" problems. With the help of the imaginary magic wand, we were able to open up space for possibilities and interactionalize the problem. The whole family, including the father, "missed" one another because of George's mandatory business trips. As a devoted husband and father, George was eventually able to negotiate with his boss a reduction in business trips. Once George started spending more time with Charlie, Charlie's behavior greatly improved. We terminated after three sessions of therapy, including the family assessment session.

Presuppositional Questions

Presuppositional questions (O'Hanlon & Weiner-Davis, 1989; Selekman, 1993) can be utilized to amplify pretreatment changes and exceptions, to convey with confidence the inevitability of change to families, to elicit the family's treatment outcome goals, and to help co-create a context for change with the family. Presuppositional questions can also produce significant changes in family members' outmoded beliefs and behaviors. In the interviewing process, we should listen carefully to individual family member's own presuppositional language and try to match our presuppositional language with theirs. For example, if the mother in a family uses past-tense presuppositional words such as "fixed" and "resolved," it makes sense for the therapist to ask questions embedded with words such as "accomplished" or "did." Like the miracle question, presuppositional questions are a powerful therapeutic tool for eliciting from family members the "who," "what," "when," "how," and "where" of goal attainment. Some examples of presuppositional questions are as follows:

"Let's say that all of you were driving home from today's session and it proved to be highly successful, what will have changed with your situation?"

"If we were to look at a videotape of this family when all of your problems are solved, what will we see happening on that video that will convince you things are better?"

"What else do we see that changed?"

"How will you know when you don't have to come here anymore?"

"I'm curious, what have you noticed that is better since you first called here to make an appointment?"

"Let's say I were to hand you my imaginary crystal ball and I asked each of you to look into the crystal ball and tell me what you see that changed over the next week with your situation?"

"How surprised will you be when that happens?" (*To identified child client*) "Which one of your parents will faint first when you do that?"

"What will be a small sign of progress over the next week that will tell you that you are really making headway?"

"How will you know that the problem is really solved?"

The following case example illustrates the therapeutic utility of presuppositional questions for co-creating a context for change with families:

Lisa, a bright 11-year-old, was school-referred for "underachieving," "not turning in her school assignments," and "talking back to her teacher." In past school years, Lisa had always received A's and B's on tests and assignments. Present in the family assessment session were Lisa; her mother, Jane; and Chester, her stepfather.

THERAPIST: Let's say I handed you my imaginary crystal ball and I asked each of you to look into the crystal ball (*all family members are staring at my hands holding the crystal ball*) and tell me what each of you see that changed over the next week with your situation?

CHESTER: Well, Lisa will be completing all of her school assignments and turning them in daily.

THERAPIST: When she does that next week, how will the two of you be getting along better?

CHESTER: Well ... I will be yelling at her less ... I know she is capable of doing better. She is a bright girl.

THERAPIST: Lisa, when Chester is yelling at you less what will he be doing instead with you that will help you guys get along better?

LISA: I would be very surprised if he would be nicer to me. I mean he is always pushing me with the schoolwork. I'm sick of it! Mom, why do you let him do that?

JANE: You know school is very important to us. Chester and I just want you to do better in school. We know you can do well if you just try. Do you really feel like we are putting too much pressure on you to do well in school?

LISA: Yes! Just leave me alone. Miss Smith [Lisa's teacher] is just like you guys. "You can do better Lisa, I know you can." That is how she sounds. That makes me mad!

THERAPIST: Lisa, please look into the imaginary crystal ball and tell me what Miss Smith is doing differently that will help the two of you get along better?

LISA: Well ... she is not trying to be my mom.

THERAPIST: What else?

LISA: She is not always asking to see my homework as soon as I walk in the door.

THERAPIST: Let's say that now I am gazing into the imaginary crystal ball, what do I see you doing differently at school that is helping you get along better with Miss Smith?

LISA: I will turn in my homework first thing. Treat her nicer. I mean not be mean to her.

THERAPIST: What about at home, what do I see you doing differently in the crystal ball with your parents?

LISA: Getting my homework done. Making sure they see I am taking it to school with me. I know what can help a lot!

THERAPIST: What?

LISA: If Mom and Chester would not push me.

THERAPIST: How so?

LISA: I will want to do my schoolwork if they leave me alone about it.

With the help of my trusty imaginary crystal ball, we were able to identify specific behaviors that maintained Lisa's difficulties with her parents, her teacher, and completing and turning in her school assignments. At the same time, by capitalizing on her own expertise, Lisa was able to identify clearly what the parents and teacher could do to resolve the difficulties. In a school meeting with the teacher, Jane, and Lisa, Lisa was able to share with her teacher that she felt as if her teacher was trying to "mother" her, which led to Lisa's "mouthing off" to Miss Smith and not doing the schoolwork. Once the parents and the teacher began to experiment with "backing off" of Lisa, particularly around her school assignments, Lisa's behavior dramatically improved. I ended up seeing the family three more times after the family assessment session.

Scaling Questions

Scaling questions (Berg & de Shazer, 1993; de Shazer, 1991, 1994) are very useful for securing a quantitative measurement of the family's presenting problem prior to treatment and presently and of where they would like to be on a scale of 1 to 10 in 1 week's time. Frequently, family members report that they have already taken constructive steps to resolve their problem situation when comparing where they were on the scale 4 weeks prior to the assessment session and where they are at presently. Like Sherlock Holmes and Miss Marple detectives, we need to elicit in great detail from each family member the useful coping and problem-solving strategies they have employed to advance themselves higher on the scale. Having family members talk about their unique creative strategies for trying to resolve the presenting problems and other difficulties empowers them and helps make it newsworthy that they are on the path to solution. Cheerleading, handshakes, and high-fives are also useful for punctuating important pretreatment changes (de Shazer, 1988, 1991; Selekman, 1993).

Once the family rates where they are on the scale presently, I ask the following question: "Let's say we get together in one week's time and you proceed to tell me that you took some steps and got to a 7 [the family was at a 6], what will you tell me that you did?" The answer to this question becomes the family's initial treatment goal, particularly if these steps are what they want to accomplish first in treatment. The therapist's job is to collaborate with the family in negotiating a solvable initial treatment goal, especially if the family's steps are too monolithic or unrealistic. Well-formed treatment goals are small, concrete, realistic, and behavioral. The therapist can ask the following kinds of questions:

> "Do you really think it is possible for your son to have a whole week without one temper tantrum, given that he has been pushed around by this problem for the past year?"

> "What will be a small sign of progress over the next week that will tell you [the parents] that we are heading in the right direction?"

> "What has to change first that will indicate that we are really succeeding here?"

> "How else will you be able to tell that we made it up to a 7 [the parent's baseline rating for their son's temper tantrum problem was a 6]?"

> "How many days out of seven will he have to go without a temper tantrum that would make you [the parents] feel like we are making good headway?"

> "On a scale from 1 to 10, with 10 being better enough, what number would you rate your situation today?"

In some cases, the therapist can establish separate goals for the child and his or her parents. This is particularly useful when the child is quite outspoken about a specific parental behavior that he or she contends is contributing to the maintenance of the difficulties. For example, if the parents' "yelling" is a major concern for the child, I may have the child rate the parents' yelling on a scale from 1 to 10, 4 weeks prior to treatment and presently. The next step for the child would be to identify as clearly as possible what the parents will need to do in a week's time to try to cut back on their yelling behavior.

Scaling questions can be used to measure family members' confidence levels regarding their ability to resolve the presenting problem. I may ask the parents to rate their confidence levels regarding their ability to resolve their son's temper tantrum problem by asking: "How confident are you today on a scale of 1 to 10 that we will resolve your son's temper tantrum problem, 10 being most confident?" With children who experience difficulty grasping the number rating process, I may use the more familiar school letter grading system (A–F) as an alternative method for eliciting a baseline measurement of his or her present behavior and to assess future progress in the goal area. Finally, with more chronic child cases, highly pessimistic parents, or families that have had multiple treatment experiences, I may reverse the scale, with 10 being the worst and 1 being the best possible rating of the presenting problem.

The following case example illustrates how scaling questions not only can pave the way for eliciting news of a difference from family members but can assist the therapist and the family in establishing a clear focus for the treatment process.

Juan was brought for therapy by his mother, Maria, because he did not follow her rules, had temper tantrums, and fought with his 8-year-old sister, Isabella. Out of respect for cultural differences, I also explored with the family how they felt about working with a non-Latino therapist. This was not a problem for them. After expanding the possibilities with the miracle question, I then asked the family scaling questions.

THERAPIST: Maria, on a scale from 1 to 10, how would you have rated Juan's behavior 4 weeks ago?

MARIA: A 2! He never listened to me. Juan used to break anything he could get his hands on when having one of his temper tantrums.

THERAPIST: What about today? How would you rate him on that scale now?

MARIA: Well . . . I think he is doing better . . . maybe he is at a 5.

THERAPIST: A 5! That's quite a leap? (*Juan is smiling in response to my reaction.*) What steps have you seen him take to get from a 2 to a 5?

MARIA: Well, we are not having no more battles about making his bed and putting his toys away. When he does have his temper fits, he is not destroying things anymore.

THERAPIST: How did you help make all of those good things happen? What are you doing differently?

MARIA: Well, I am more patient. I am not yelling as much. You know what really works?

THERAPIST: What?

MARIA: Avoiding the power struggles.

THERAPIST: How did you come up with that great idea?

MARIA: Well, before ... I used to try and win the battles by screaming and taking away everything ... but that only made the situation worse.

THERAPIST: Are there other things that you are doing that helps?

MARIA: When Juan has had a good week, I reward him by taking him out for pizza and a movie.

THERAPIST: Wow! You are really creative as a parent. What is your consultation fee? I want to use you as an expert consultant with some of my other single-parent family cases (*laughing*).

MARIA: It's been hard raising these two kids, but I keep telling myself, "You're going to make it ... "

THERAPIST: (*looking at Juan*) What is your mom doing now that helps the most, so that you don't get into trouble?

JUAN: She is not yelling. Pizza and movies (*smiling and hugging his mother*)!

THERAPIST: What do you like on your pizza?

JUAN: Lots of sausage and cheese!

THERAPIST: Maria, let's say we were to get together in a week and you proceed to tell me that Juan took some further steps to get up to a 6! What will you tell me he did to get to a 6?

MARIA: He won't be fighting as much with his sister.

THERAPIST: What will be a small sign of progress over the next week that will tell you we are making headway with the fighting situation?

MARIA: Rather than punching his sister when she teases him or makes him mad, he will come to me instead.

THERAPIST: Do you think it is realistic that he will be able to do that everyday?

MARIA: No, probably not.

THERAPIST: How many days over the next week would you be happy with?

MARIA: If he could do this twice I would be thrilled!

THERAPIST: *(looking at Juan)* Do you think you can pull that off?

JUAN: Yeah. I want pizza!

I ended up seeing Juan and his family three times. Juan had a great week in that he only fought with his sister once and had no temper tantrums. The added bonus in this case was working with a mother who was so committed, creative, and resourceful as a parent that it made my job easy. There were also a wealth of pretreatment changes to amplify and consolidate.

COLLABORATIVE TREATMENT PLANNING

Once the family's initial treatment goals have been negotiated, the therapist needs to share with the family the modalities and methods he or she will use to help the family rapidly achieve their goals. The unique needs of each case determine how future family therapy sessions will be structured. If it appears that it would be most advantageous to divide up the session time into three parts (seeing the whole family together for a time, meeting with the parents without the children present, and seeing the identified child alone), I explore with the family whether they think this session format can be useful to them. I let the family know that they will be offered tasks or experiments to perform between our visits to help get the "change ball rolling." I like to stress to families that most of their changes will occur outside my office. Finally, I like to share with families that they will be in the driver's seat in terms of determining the frequency of visits and that I will recommend vacations from counseling as a vote of confidence to them once there is progress.

When multiple helping professionals from larger systems are involved with the family, I invite the family to tell me with whom I need to collaborate. I secure signed consent forms from the family to collaborate with all these key members of the problem system. As part of the macrosystemic assessment process (Selekman, 1993), I explore with the family whether there are any concerned relatives or significant others with whom I should collaborate or who should be actively involved in the treatment process as well. I share with the family the importance of our collaboration with these involved helpers so as to maximize opportunities for them to hear about the changes they are making in counseling. It is also helpful to explore with the family whether they need the therapist to advocate for them in helping resolve impasses with other community agencies and to assist in getting information about particular community resources.

If a child comes to the family assessment session already on prescribed medications, I have the parents sign a consent form so I can collaborate with the pediatrician or psychiatrist involved with the medication management process. Although I have a lot of concerns about the use of psychotropic medications on children because of some of the side effects, some children greatly benefit from a combination of family therapy and low dosages of medication (Barkley, 1995; Barkley, Guevremont, Anastopoulos, & Fletcher, 1992)

When selecting a DSM-IV Axis I diagnosis for the identified child client for insurance purposes, I like to involve the family in the decision-making process. If the child's diagnosis could be one of three possibilities, I show the family the DSM-IV descriptions for each of the diagnostic categories and have them pick the one they think best fits their situation. Many children's problems are some form of an adjustment disorder, so I often give the family a grand tour of this section of DSM-IV. When in doubt, we may go with the adjustment disorder, not otherwise specified label. Because many insurance companies do not accept V codes, we are often forced to select an Axis I diagnosis for the identified client even though the truth of the matter is that we are dealing with a family problem. When families are wedded to a particular Axis I DSM-IV diagnostic label, I go with their label initially and work with it in the treatment process, often by externalizing the problem (Selekman, 1996; White & Epston, 1990).

In a similar collaborative fashion, I invite the family to be coauthors in writing any treatment updates and summaries and letters for involved helpers from larger systems, the court, schools, and managed care companies. By doing this, we empower families to be in charge of their destinies.

THE EDITORIAL REFLECTION

Approximately 45 minutes into the hour, I take an intersession break to compose my editorial reflection for the family. The editorial consists of positively relabeled problem behaviors, normalizing concerns, compliments for each family member on the various problem-solving and coping strategies they reported engaging in that were helpful to them, questions to think about regarding their situation, and a therapeutic task or experiments to test that fit with the unique cooperative response patterns of each family member.

When complimenting family members, it is important to carefully gauge where each member is in terms of optimism, pessimism, and customership. For instance, if the therapist showers highly pessimistic complainant-type parents and their child with too many positively toned compliments, the parents may think the therapist is being sarcastic or not taking their situation serious enough. The same is true with too much positive relabeling: More pessimistic family members may think the therapist is trying to talk them out of their problems.

While composing the editorial reflection, if there are certain elements of the family's story about which I am curious, I share with the family my questions as part of the reflection process. I begin my questions with qualifiers as "I wonder if . . . " or "Could it be . . . ?" Sometimes I leave the family with some questions to think about when concluding the session and do not offer them a task or experiments. The care of Lisa and her family provides a clinical illustration of using questions in the editorial reflection portion of the session (see pp. 61–63). I asked them the following questions I was pondering:

> "I wondered how it was decided that Chester be in charge of monitoring Lisa's schoolwork?"

> "Could it be that this is a tough spot for a new step-parent to be in?"

> "I wondered if Lisa and Chester would be getting along better if he did not have this responsibility?"

By asking such questions, therapists convey to the families that the therapist is not a privileged expert on their problem situation and that the therapeutic process is collaborative. The questions can also open up space for possibilities.

When engaging in the editorial reflection, it is most important to utilize the family members' language and speak to their beliefs about themselves and their problem story. By doing this, any new ideas offered or tasks prescribed are more likely to be acceptable to the family. There are two advantages to taking an intersession break 10–15 minutes prior to the end of the hour: (1) The therapist has time to compose a thoughtful editorial reflection as well as select or construct therapeutic tasks that fit with the unique cooperative response patterns of family members, and (2) family members are more than likely sitting on the edge of their seats wondering what the therapist has to say about them. Families that have had past negative experiences with therapists are usually surprised to be complimented on their strengths and resources and to be working with a therapist who appears to be trying very hard to understand their problem story and to help navigate them in the direction of change.

POST-ASSESSMENT SESSION SELF-REFLECTION

Following the family assessment session, I like to set aside a little time to reflect on my therapeutic actions in the session and my clinical impressions and formulations of the case. As questions and ideas pop into my mind, I write them down as a checklist for future thinking and pathways to pursue with a case. I divide my self-reflection process into two different areas: (1) reflection on action taken in the session and areas to explore with the family and (2) alternative therapeutic actions to pursue in the next family session. With reflection-on-action taken, I may ask myself the following questions:

> "If I were to conduct this session all over again with this same family, what would I do differently?"

> "What should I ask them more about?"

> "Do I know what they perceive as the 'real' problem?"

> "Should I use less or more humor with this family?"

> "What family member strengths and resources did I fail to capitalize on?"

> "Who responded the best to being complimented?"

> "Who responded the least to the compliments?"

> "What family members do I need to spend more time engaging in the next session?"

> "What other tasks could I have given family members that might have better fit with their unique cooperative response patterns?"

When thinking about my clinical impressions and formulation of the case, I may ask myself the following questions:

> "Do we have a customer here?"

"If not, who should I try and engage for future sessions?"

"What involved helping professionals at the school are part of the problem system?"

"What else am I curious about with this case?"

"I wonder if the parent's goal is still too monolithic?"

"If we renegotiated their goal into more solvable terms, what would that look like?"

"What are the key solution-building patterns?"

"What are the patterns that connect?"

"Have I been sensitive to cultural issues?"

"Are there power imbalances around gender in this family?"

With second and subsequent sessions, the same critical self-reflective process can be utilized to monitor our clinical thinking and therapeutic actions closely with each family with which we work. By viewing ourselves in relationship to our clients through a critical lens, we can remain therapeutically flexible, maintain a kaleidoscopic view of families, and carefully tailor what we say or do to the uniqueness of each family.

CHAPTER 3

Interviewing for Change: Questions as Interventive Tools for Empowering Children and Their Families

Leading the patient to "See what I (the patient) can
do," is much more effective than letting the patient see
what things the therapist can do with or to the patient.
                                        –MILTON H. ERICKSON

In the quote above, Erickson is referring to a technique that is at the heart of interviewing for change. Inviting families to talk about their past successes, their strengths, and where they want to be when they have an ideal outcome empowers them to create their own positive self-fulfilling prophecies. Questions can be used as interventive tools for promoting self-healing, challenging outmoded family beliefs, and sparking curiosity, which can lead to possibilities for stuck families. The quality of the learning process for families depends on the quality of the questions we ask. Bold and intriguing questions that elicit a full range of responses are more likely to open up space for new learning and the emergence of creative solutions with families (Brown & Isaacs, 1997).

In this chapter, I present five interventive questions that can be utilized at any stage of family treatment. Family members' unique cooperative response patterns, the age of the child, and the nature of the family's presenting problem dictate which categories of questions will be used in the interviewing process. Unlike the conversational (Anderson & Goolishian, 1988b) and goal-setting questions described in Chapter 2, the five questions described in this chapter are particularly useful for challenging rigid family beliefs and moving the treatment system (therapist and family) out of an impasse situation. Children also tend to respond well to questions that draw upon their creativity and expertise, such as the imagination and reversal questions presented later in this chapter.

INTERVIEWING FOR CHANGE

The Solution-Oriented therapist asks questions in a purposeful manner, by carefully assessing family members' unique cooperative response patterns and matching questions with those patterns (de Shazer, 1988, 1991, 1994; Lipchik, 1988; O'Hanlon & Weiner-Davis, 1989). The purposeful interview is a circular process in which family members' verbal and nonverbal feedback guides the therapist toward future question category selection. For example, if I ask the miracle question (de Shazer, 1988) and, in the middle of the miracle inquiry, a family member has a concern he or she wishes to address, I shift into more open-ended conversational questions (Andersen, 1991; Anderson & Goolishian, 1988a, 1988b) to address his or her concerns and make room for storytelling. Once the family member's concerns have been adequately addressed, the therapist can move back to the miracle question inquiry and invite other family members to share their ideal miracle pictures. The Solution-Oriented therapists must, like ballet dancers, be flexible and on their toes, ready to move in any direction family members wish to take them. If the therapist finds a particular category of questions that appears verbally and nonverbally to be creating possibilities with family members, it is most advantageous to do more of what's working with the family. Finally, when interviewing children, it is important for the therapist to concretize his or her language and to use words that the child can grasp intellectually.

Five different categories of interventive questions, followed here by guidelines for question category selection and case illustrations, demonstrate the utility of the various interventive questions in the interviewing process.

Imagination Questions

Developmentally, children begin displaying signs of imaginative play and pretending after 1½ years of age. Parents can help cultivate their children's abilities to engage in imaginative play by modeling make-believe play. Research indicates that very imaginative children tend to be better at concentrating, developing creative solutions to problems, and displaying good self-control (Schaefer & DiGeronimo, 1995). The stage of development a child is at dictates the level of sophistication the therapist's imagination questions and scenarios can be. For example, we know that 3- to 6-year-olds have vivid fantasy lives and are at the peak of their ability to pretend and use their imagination abilities (Schaefer & DiGeronimo, 1995). Imagination questions fit nicely with children's developmental need to dramatize their social worlds through play and pretending.

Before selecting the type of imagination questions I want to use with a particular child and his or her family, I first assess the following: What are the child's favorite TV, movie, and book characters? What are the child's favorite pastimes, hobbies, and talents? Who are the child's favorite music stars? If the child could be someone famous in history, in the music world, on TV, or a book character for a day, who would the child want to be, and why? If the child could choose one TV show in which he or she would like to star, which TV show would he or she select? What role would he or she play and why? If the child created his or her own TV show about the family, what would the show be about? Such questions can help spark creativity in both the therapist and the child when collaborating for solutions in the interviewing process. Because using imagination and pretending fits so nicely with children's worlds, they typically warm up to and enjoy when therapists tap into their natural creative abilities. Through the use of imagination questions, therapy sessions become more fun and adventurous for children and their families.

> Marci, a 4-year-old, was brought for therapy by her mother for "power struggles" around bedtime and for "night terrors," which were diagnosed by their pediatrician. Except for this time of the day, Marci reportedly was highly "cooperative," "friendly," not anxious, and "a pleasure to be around." According to the mother, Melinda, Marci's preschool teacher consistently found Marci to be a "real joy" in class. Marci was an only child, but her mother described her as being very sociable and having friends in the neighborhood. In exploring with Marci what her favorite TV shows were, she shared with me that she liked "Barney" a lot. I noticed that Marci brought with her a purse with Baby Bop illustrations on it. Because Marci appeared to be a Barney fan club member, I decided to capitalize on her fondness for Barney in the interviewing process.

THERAPIST: Marci, let's say your mother turned on the Barney show for you tomorrow and we saw Marci on the show. We saw you as a friend visiting Barney and Baby Bop. You came to see Barney and Baby Bop to find out if they could help you go to sleep when you have to go to bed. What would Barney say to help you on TV?

MARCI: Barney would hug me; tell me, "Don't be scared."

THERAPIST: Would Barney say anything else to you?

MARCI: I don't know . . .

THERAPIST: Do you think Barney might say, "Most girls and boys get scared when they go to sleep, but it will go away"?

MARCI: Yeah.

THERAPIST: What do you think, Melinda? Do you think Barney would say that to Marci?

MELINDA: Yes! And I think Barney would tell her this "will go away." "Don't be scared."

THERAPIST: Marci, what do you think Baby Bop would tell you?

MARCI: She would be nice to me; hug me; tell me, "It's okay . . . I'm your friend."

THERAPIST: What would Barney and Baby Bop do with you on TV to help you?

MARCI: Sing me songs. Watch me when I sleep so I'm not scared.

THERAPIST: So, on TV we would see Barney and Baby Bop in your bedroom standing over you to help you sleep? Does that help?

MARCI: Yeah. I'm sleeping. Barney will say, "Remember, I love you!"

Based on the success of these questions in eliciting images of Marci's receiving support from Barney and Baby Bop with the sleeping problem, the mother and I designed a nighttime ritual in which she and her daughter would carry her stuffed Barney and Baby Bop dolls from the playroom into her bedroom prior to going to bed. Marci would then hug each one of the stuffed dolls and place them in toddler-sized chairs that she would position around her bed. Not only did this ritual eliminate the power struggle problem, it had a profound impact on the night terror difficulty as well.

Resiliency Questions

Family members' resiliencies are our main allies in the solution-construction process. Having family members talk about their past successes, how they triumphed over crisis and adversity, can offer therapists important clues about potential problem-solving and coping strategies to capitalize on and channel into the presenting problem area. Families are often surprised when they are asked about their strengths. Families that have experienced failure in previous treatment can be empowered by a therapeutic focus on their competency areas and what is "right" about them.

At times, I have the family describe themselves in detail as a group successfully mastering a past crisis situation as if they were watching a videotape. I use this videotape of mastery as a guide to help them resolve the current presenting problem. Similarly, I may have athletic children use a hypothetical videotape of themselves in the past performing with excellence in a sporting event and have them visualize the video to cope with current stressors. It is also quite helpful to have parents share with the identified child client what they did as children to cope with or to resolve similar difficulties.

> George, 10 years old, was brought for therapy by his mother, Elizabeth, for somatic complaints, such as "headaches" and a "nervous stomach," and some decline in school performance. Elizabeth also thought that George might be "depressed." George was an only child. His parents had been separated for more than 1 year because of his father's severe alcoholism problem. George had been having a hard time for the past 3 years coping with his father's "arguing" with his mother and "passing out on the floor in his vomit" after being highly intoxicated and all the "forgotten promises." George had been receiving some supportive counseling at his school. George had infrequent contacts with his father, who had moved out of state. The father, Bill, had been through four inpatient treatment experiences for alcoholism, all unsuccessful. Inevitably, he would start drinking again a few weeks after being discharged. Because this family had experienced so much emotional pain and suffering, I was curious about their resiliencies, what was keeping them going? How did they bounce back after a crisis with the father? I invited the family to share with me what they viewed as their strengths.
>
> THERAPIST: I am amazed how resilient you guys are, in terms of what you have been through together and how you keep

pushing ahead. What's your secret? I mean I've worked with a lot of families that have been oppressed by alcoholism problems for years, just like yours, and their situations were a lot worse. What are your family strengths, so I can teach other families the tools that work?

ELIZABETH: Well, George and I have really pulled closer together. I really try and be there for him. He knows (*looking at George*) that I really love him and will always be there for him.

THERAPIST: Besides being there for support, what other strengths do the two of you have?

ELIZABETH: He is a big help in the kitchen.

THERAPIST: George, what are your house specialties? I mean, what do you like to cook? (*Both laugh.*)

GEORGE: Well, I can make eggs, macaroni and cheese . . . peanut butter and jelly sandwiches.

THERAPIST: Wow! How did you learn how to make all of those dishes?

ELIZABETH: He's really a good cook. We also bake chocolate chip cookies together.

THERAPIST: Elizabeth, I want to go back in time for a few minutes. Can you think of other things you used to do when Bill was in the home to help George weather the storm after a crisis situation, like Bill's passing out or after witnessing you guys arguing?

ELIZABETH: I would take him into his bedroom and tell him, "It's not your fault"; "We love you"; "Only Daddy can decide to stop drinking, we can't stop his drinking."

THERAPIST: Does that seem to help?

ELIZABETH: I think, sometimes. George loves his father and really misses him.

THERAPIST: George, when Mom used to do those things, were they helpful?

GEORGE: Yeah, I guess . . .

THERAPIST: Anything she did or is still doing that helps you deal with your dad's drinking?

GEORGE: Well, telling me that I can't stop my dad's drinking. I like when she hugs me when I'm upset.

THERAPIST: Anything else?

GEORGE: No. Mom, can I go get a pop? (*Elizabeth gives him money to buy a soft drink.*)

THERAPIST: Elizabeth, if somebody stopped you on the street and asked you, "What are your strengths as a family?", what would you say?

ELIZABETH: We are loving, very close, and we manage to do fun things, despite all of the problems.

THERAPIST: How about three adjectives to describe your family?

ELIZABETH: Courageous, strong, and bright. What should I do about George's headaches and stomachaches?

THERAPIST: Have they been medically checked?

ELIZABETH: Yes, the pediatrician could not find anything. He thinks it's stress. (*George returns with his Coke.*) What do you think?

THERAPIST: It sounds like, George, you have had to stomach a lot with your dad's passing out, being drunk, and when your parents used to argue. George, this is going to sound like a strange question but, if your stomach could talk to us about what's been going on with you and your family, what would it say? (*George smiles and laughs.*)

GEORGE: (*looking at his mother, smiling*) You're right . . . that's a weird question.

THERAPIST: Just play around with it . . . pretend your stomach could talk to us.

GEORGE: Well . . . it hurts, I guess . . . "Stop making me hurt."

THERAPIST: Would it say anything else?

GEORGE: I don't know what else . . .

THERAPIST: "Stop making me hurt." Do you think your stomach is trying to tell you and your mom something?

GEORGE: I'm not sure.

ELIZABETH: Maybe the stomach is trying to tell us that we are hurting, both of us because of all of the problems, you know, the drinking situation.

THERAPIST: What do you think, George?

GEORGE: I don't know . . . maybe.

By inviting family members to talk about their resiliencies and past successes, we can learn about what coping strategies we need to mobilize and increase in frequency to help this family resolve their current difficulties. Elizabeth's resiliencies of parental optimism, emotional support, and good problem-solving abilities were instrumental in helping George through some rough times. George's key protective factors for coping were his intelligence, good problem-solving abilities, and seeking his mother's emotional support in times of trouble. I also had the family construct a Victory Box to serve as a constant reminder of their resilience and creative problem-solving abilities.

When clients are oppressed by somatic problems, I have found it most advantageous to invite the client to put a voice to the affected body part. Not only does it externalize the problem (White, 1995), but it helps challenge outmoded beliefs about the somatic complaint because family members begin to see it as a metaphor for the family drama. I used a similar strategy with George's headache problem. We were quickly able to stabilize the presenting problems by using this therapeutic strategy and capitalizing on family members' resiliencies.

Reversal Questions

In my clinical work with children and their families, I like to utilize the children as expert consultants in the interviewing process. For some therapists, it may seem illogical to invite children to give their parents advice on parenting and problem solving. However, I have been consistently impressed with how bright, insightful, and creative children are when it comes to solving family problems. When asked, children clearly spell out what specific parental behaviors contribute to the maintenance of the presenting problems and are eager to share with their parents what they can do that can lead to problem resolution. While at their friends' houses, children often learn through observation and carefully listening to what their friends' parents do what seems to work in their relationships. Children care about their parent's well-being and often have some good ideas about what their parents can do to help reduce some of the stress in their lives.

By utilizing children as expert consultants in the treatment process, therapists can strengthen their therapeutic alliance with the child, give the child a "voice" in the problem-solving effort, and challenge the parents' unhelpful beliefs about the identified child client. Reversal questions can help interactionalize the problem. Finally, actively involving the child in the solution construction process can greatly reduce lengths of stay in treatment.

Nadia, 10 years old, was brought for therapy by her parents for "emotional problems" related to her chronic difficulties with asthma. The parents came from Brazil but Nadia was born in the United States. The father was a successful pilot. Sylvia, the mother, "did not work," had only "one friend," and spent most of her leisure time "taking care of" and entertaining Nadia. Nadia was their "special child," for Sylvia lost three babies through miscarriages. Fernando was away a lot on international flights. The parents reported that they almost lost Nadia twice to severe asthma attacks. Sylvia, sitting right next to Nadia, got very emotional when reminiscing about how they almost lost their daughter. The presenting problems with Nadia were temper tantrums, not putting her belongings away, and limit testing with the mother. Because Nadia was an extremely bright and precocious child, I decided to use her as a co-therapist and find out whether she had any advice for the parents that could help improve things at home.

THERAPIST: We have been talking a lot about your [the parents] concern with Nadia. It sounds like Sylvia that you're with Nadia the most, is that right?

SYLVIA: Yes. Fernando does not have to deal with Nadia during the week because he is away most of the time.

THERAPIST: Since we have not heard much from Nadia and she is such a bright girl, I would like to borrow your [Nadia] brain for a few minutes. Nadia, do you have any advice for your mother that can help you get along better?

NADIA: She worries too much. Mom is always asking me, "Did you take your medicine?" "Where is your inhaler?" It makes me mad. She doesn't trust me.

FERNANDO: Nadia, are there not times that you have forgot to take your medicine and the inhaler to school?

NADIA: Yes, but not a lot.

THERAPIST: Nadia, do you have any advice for your mother that can help her worry less about you?

NADIA: Go out with Yolanda [mother's friend] more. Mom sits around the house too much.

THERAPIST: What else do you [Nadia] think your mother should be doing instead of sitting around the house?

NADIA: Go to the mall. Maybe work again ... remember, Mom, you used to work at that clothing store?

SYLVIA: You're right, honey. I should get out more. I just worry a lot about you ...

THERAPIST: It is obvious to me that you [Sylvia] have a big heart and that you and Fernando have done a super job with Nadia. Thanks a lot, Nadia, for all your good advice. Listen, if I have any problem with my 3-year-old daughter can I consult with you? (*Everyone laughs.*)

Nadia's expert advice proved to be instrumental in helping create more breathing room in her relationship with her mother. Sylvia, in particular, had not heard Nadia's concerns before, so this was a newsworthy experience for her. Sylvia eventually secured a part-time job and made a few friends at work. Once Sylvia was less vigilant around Nadia, Nadia's behavior greatly improved, especially in taking her medication and carrying the inhaler around with her. In a later therapy session, I helped Sylvia mourn the losses of her three babies. These painful losses and nearly losing Nadia twice to asthma attacks had kept Sylvia stuck in terms of taking care of her own needs outside of motherhood.

Future-Oriented Questions

When the treatment system is stuck, or we are working with "past-bound" (Tomm, 1987), chronic, or entrenched families, future-oriented questions can be utilized to help create possibilities. The great psychoanalyst Harry Stack Sullivan's core belief was that "the basic direction of the human organism is forward." Sullivan always approached his patients with an optimistic stance. Sullivan said the following:

Thirty years of work has taught me that, whenever one could be aided to foresee the reasonable probability of a better future, everyone will show a sufficient tendency to collaborate in the achievement of more adequate and appropriate ways of living. (cited in Cottrell & Foote, 1995, p. 203)

Having families envision a future place in time in which they have realized their desired outcomes can be a liberating experience for them, particularly when they are feeling so paralyzed by their presenting problems. The future becomes the now for the family. According to cognitive researcher Palmarini (1994), "The easier it is to imagine an event or a situation, and the more the occurrence impresses us emotionally, the more likely we are to think of it as also objectively frequent" (p. 128). With the help of future-oriented questions, we can co-create with families positive self-fulfilling prophecies.

> Cody, 9 years old, was reluctantly brought for therapy (by his parents) for "stealing," "beating on" his 8-year-old sister, engaging in power struggles, and "not following the rules." Cody was having behavioral "problems in school" as well. The parents were very pessimistic and frustrated by Cody's chronic behavioral problems. After three previous treatment failures with psychologists, the parents were not very hopeful that our treatment experience together would be any different. It was quite clear in the session that there was a lot of conflict between Cody and his father, Dan. Dan reprimanded Cody twice in our session for antagonizing his sister, Tiffany. When I asked the miracle question (de Shazer, 1988), the parents and the children responded with more pessimism. The more I tried to cooperate with the family's pessimism, the more pessimistic they became. At this point in the session I shifted gears and decided to ask future-oriented questions to try to move the family and myself in a different direction. Present in the family interview were Cody, Tiffany, Dan, and Rachel, the mother.

> THERAPIST: Let's say that I ran into you guys at a 7-Eleven 6 months down the road, long after we successfully completed counseling together, and I asked all of you what steps you took to get out of counseling, what will you tell me you did?

> RACHEL: I would tell you that Cody is cooperative, we are no longer fighting about everything, and he is playing in a nicer way with Tiffany.

> THERAPIST: What effect had all of those changes had on your relationship with Cody?

> RACHEL: We're getting along better. I am taking him out more to the mall. You know, doing things that he likes to do.

THERAPIST: What else will you tell me that you are doing differently as parents that is now helping you and Cody get along better?

DAN: Avoiding power struggles. Not being so reactive to little things that Cody does.

THERAPIST: What difference has that made when you are doing that?

DAN: Less battles. Less stress.

RACHEL: I like him more when he is not being so difficult.

THERAPIST: What about you Cody, what will you tell me that is better with your parents when I see you guys at 7-Eleven?

CODY: They are not yelling at me. We are not fighting. Daddy's playing video games with me.

THERAPIST: Cody, if your teacher popped into 7-Eleven right now, what will she tell me you are doing good in her class?

CODY: I'm paying attention, not getting into fights . . . doing my work.

THERAPIST: Will she tell me that she is not missing things from her desktop anymore?

CODY: Yeah . . . I don't take things anymore.

By using future-oriented questions, we were able to open up the door for possibilities. For the first time in the family interview, family members began sharing creative problem-solving strategies that they believed could work in improving their situation. While sharing their unique solutions, they spoke about the changes in past tense, as if they already happened. The future became the now, which liberated the family from feeling stuck in the present. The added bonus for myself was that I no longer felt stuck therapeutically, thanks to the family's guiding me in the direction of change.

Externalizing the Problem

Families that have experienced multiple treatment failures and have been oppressed by their problems for a long time tend to be very demoralized and stuck by the time of our initial contact with them. Some of these families will be hard-pressed to identify any newsworthy pretreatment changes or past successes that we can capitalize on to empower them. Therefore, externalizing their oppressive presenting problem (White, 1995; White & Epston, 1990) may be a viable therapeutic option to pursue when solution-oriented questions are eliciting information from family members that does not make a difference in altering their outmoded beliefs. When externalizing the problem, it is crucial for the therapist to co-construct a new description of the problem that is based on the family's beliefs about their difficulty and the language they use to describe it. Therapists can be as creative as they wish with what they externalize the problem into (e.g., ADD and other DSM-IV labels), particularly with parents who are wedded to the labels with which they come in the door; lying, fears, and other problematic behaviors; the "attitude"; habits; the temper; "arguing"; "blaming"; problem lifestyles; and so forth.

Externalizing the problem is a two-step process:

1. Map the influence the problem has over the identified client, family members, and significant others (peers, relatives, and involved helping professionals).

2. Map the influence the identified client, family members, and significant others have over the problem.

The first step of the process is to explore the effects the problem has had on family members' self-perceptions and relationships with each other and others (White, 1995). A family pushed around by the identified client's "attitude" problem can be asked: "How long has the 'attitude' been pushing all of you around for?" "What does the 'attitude' brainwash Billy to do?" Such questions help deconstruct fixed family beliefs about the identified client's behavior and convey the idea to the family that they are all, including the identified client, being victimized by the presenting problem.

The second category of questions is critical for the restorying process as the questions pave the way for the creation of an alternative family story. Story lines of competency or unique outcomes (White, 1995) are elicited from family members to create a double description of the family's original problem-saturated story. Unique outcome questions (White, 1988) elicit from family members times when they have stood up to or fighting back against the oppressive problem rather than succumbing to its powerful influence on them. Some examples of unique account questions are as follows: "I'm curious, Steve, have there been any times lately where you tricked 'lying' and you didn't allow it to get you into trouble with your parents?" "Can you think of a time lately where the Temper was lurking about, but you guys [the parents] stood your ground and didn't allow it to divide you?" As part of the restorying process, White (1995) stresses the importance of incorporating an "audience" of involved and concerned others in the lives of the identified client and the family to contribute to the newly developing alternative family story and to help "authenticate" it.

> Johnny, 10 years old, was school-referred for ADD, being highly "disruptive" in class, and "not following the rules" at home. Johnny's mother, Barbara, was remarried and had three other children from her second marriage. His biological parents had divorced when Johnny was 6. Johnny had regular weekly contact with his natural father. According to Barbara, Johnny had always been in special education programs because of his behavioral difficulties. The parents had also taken Johnny to a "special ADD clinic" where he received several "batteries of tests" that "proved he had ADD." They had seen four other therapists before me. Barbara, Warren (the stepfather), and Johnny described the ADD problem as being oppressive and chronic. I decided to externalize the problem (White, 1995; White & Epston, 1990) because the mother, stepfather, and Johnny were so pessimistic and paralyzed by the wrath of ADD. Present in the first family interview were Barbara, Warren, and Johnny.

THERAPIST: How long has ADD been pushing all of you around for?

BARBARA: Three years.

THERAPIST: When ADD is getting the best of Johnny, what sort of things does it make him do?

BARBARA: Well, he is aggravating Ann [7 years old], he doesn't listen to me . . . I tell him to put his things away and he tells me to "shut up." Boy, does he got a mouth on him!

THERAPIST: Does ADD make him swear at you?

BARBARA: Yeah . . . and it's sort of strange but I can tell that he's getting an ADD attack when he gets all wound up, swears, and doesn't listen.

THERAPIST: What about you, Warren. Does ADD coach Johnny to push your buttons as well?

WARREN: Yes! I always have to scream at him a few times before he does what I want him to do.

BARBARA: Yeah, sometimes it is like talking to the wall. The child gets taken over by this ADD thing . . .

THERAPIST: So ADD brainwashes him to get out of control or does it invade his body like an evil spirit?

BARBARA: Warren, wouldn't you say it was like an evil spirit?

WARREN: Yes. He gets mad and mouthy and very difficult to manage.

THERAPIST: When ADD is getting the best of you parents, what does it make the two of you do?

WARREN: We argue a lot about how to manage him. I think she is too lenient. I'm more the screamer.

BARBARA: I don't like when Warren screams so much. So to try and keep things calm, I let Johnny off the hook ... I know it's wrong ... but I don't know ... I feel frustrated.

THERAPIST: So ADD divides the two of you? Do both of you feel frustrated by what ADD is doing to this family?

WARREN: Yes, I feel frustrated too. This ADD thing has made our life hell! We can't leave Johnny alone with Ann.

THERAPIST: Johnny, what does ADD coach you to do in class?

JOHNNY: I fight. I don't listen to the teacher. I get mad a lot.

THERAPIST: Does ADD ever make you feel dumb?

JOHNNY: Yeah (*looking sad*).

THERAPIST: What else does ADD try and teach you about yourself?

JOHNNY: I'm not a good boy. I can't do the work.

After mapping the influence that ADD had over individual family members and family relationships, I shifted gears to begin the restorying process by mapping the influence that Johnny, his parents, and the teacher had over ADD. I attempted to elicit story lines of competency and examples of the family protesting against ADD's reigning over them.

THERAPIST: Warren and Barbara, can you think of anything that you guys have done in the past to stand up to ADD and not allowed it to get the best of Johnny?

BARBARA: Not yelling a lot. He seems to calm down faster when we don't scream at him.

WARREN: I agree, but it also helps if we work together. You've got to stop giving in to him. You know that makes me mad.

THERAPIST: So, if you guys cut back on the yelling and don't let ADD divide you, it seems to help?

WARREN: Yes, definitely.

BARBARA: He's right . . . I need to be tougher with him.

THERAPIST: Can you think of other things you have done to not allow ADD to back Johnny into a corner?

BARBARA: No . . . not that I can think of.

THERAPIST: How about you Johnny, when ADD is trying to get you into trouble with your parents, can you think of anything they do that helps you out?

JOHNNY: Not yelling. Not fighting. When we are happy.

THERAPIST: What do you do as a family that makes you happy?

JOHNNY: We play video games. Warren takes us to the baseball game.

THERAPIST: What about at school, does Miss Johnson [the teacher] do anything to stop ADD from pushing you around?

JOHNNY: She is not always yelling at me. She's nicer. She sees that I'm trying to do my work.

By the end of the session, the parents and Johnny were viewing ADD as the real villain. The parents began to interact with Johnny in a more positive manner. Once the parents and the teacher stopped their "yelling" and became more of a unified "team," Johnny's behavior dramatically improved. Johnny's view of himself as being an incompetent "bad boy" changed as well. After six sessions over a 6-month period, the label ADD was no longer being used to describe Johnny's behavior, and he was mainstreamed back to a regular classroom setting by the end of the school year. Although the school was being cautious about mainstreaming Johnny too quickly, he displayed a great deal of patience and he continued to prove the skeptics wrong by pioneering a new direction with his school career.

CONCLUSION

In this chapter, I have presented a variety of pathways that therapists can pursue in the interviewing process with families. With the help of interventive questions, families can offer therapists valuable feedback about how to better cooperate with them and important clues about what and how they want to change. Finally, interviewing for change can help inform therapeutic task design and selection.

CHAPTER 4

Finding Fit: Guidelines for Therapeutic Task Design, Selection, and Implementation

Yes, therapy should always be designed to fit the
patient and not the patient to fit the therapy.
                        –MILTON H. ERICKSON

When selecting and designing therapeutic tasks for children and their
families, there are four important elements to consider: (1) the family's
definition of the problem; (2) key family member characteristics, that
is, language, beliefs, strengths to utilize; (3) the unique cooperative
response patterns of family members; and (4) the family's treatment
goals. Unless we make careful use of these important elements, any
therapeutic task we select or design may fail to *fit* (de Shazer, 1985)
for family members and may lead to their feeling misunderstood,
lacking confidence in our ability to help, and possibly dropping out of
treatment.

After a brief discussion of each of the key elements in the
therapeutic task selection and construction process, I will present five
idea-generating strategies that can aid therapists in designing creative
therapeutic tasks. The final section of this chapter elaborates on three
Solution-Focused Therapy tasks that can be quite effective with specific
types of child case situations.

THE KEY ELEMENTS FOR OPTIMIZING FIT WITH THERAPEUTIC TASK DESIGN AND SELECTION

According to problem-solving expert and researcher Arthur Van Gundy, "We must know where we are before we can begin the journey to where we want to be" (1988, p. 19). Therefore, we need to make sure with our clients not only that we have selected the "right" problem to work on but that it is well-defined. We can determine the "right" problem with our clients by having them prioritize and clarify which aspect or part of the presenting problem they would like to resolve first. A well-defined and negotiated problem is specific, behavioral, and solvable. For example, a mother brought in her 6-year-old boy for treatment because she felt he had a "low self-esteem" problem. Upon further questioning and in an effort to negotiate low self-esteem into solvable terms, the mother reported that it was her son's "temper tantrum" problem that was the real problem she wanted help with. Because temper tantrum problems are behavioral and much more solvable than low self-esteem problems, we were quickly able to resolve this problem.

The true master and creator of the utilization strategy in psychotherapy was Milton H. Erickson. Erickson would utilize whatever his clients brought to therapy, which included key words and beliefs, life themes, metaphors, nonverbals, verbal communication, style, talents, interests, and hobbies (Erickson & Rossi, 1983; Gordon & Meyers-Anderson, 1981). As part of the engagement process, I like to spend ample time finding out from each family member what their strengths, talents, and hobbies are. With children, I like to carefully observe what toys, books, and art media attract their attention the most and the nature of their play style so that I can use these things in both the engagement process and the therapeutic task selection and design. When inquiring about the family's presenting problems, I listen carefully to the words family members use to describe their problems, their beliefs about why the problems are occurring, and any key family themes or metaphors. Asking "why" questions serves as a direct pipeline into family members' beliefs about the causation of the presenting problems and provides important clues for determining the real problem with the family. Parents may be asked, "What's your theory about why this problem is happening?" Once we gain access to what the family believes is the real problem, we can use their key words, beliefs, family themes, metaphors, and strengths when constructing and offering them a therapeutic task as an experiment. The following case example illustrates the utilization strategy with therapeutic task design.

Catherine brought her 10-year-old son, Dylan, and 11-year-old son, Jaime, for therapy for constantly "mouthing off" to her and "refusing to do their chores" and comply with her "rules." Catherine had divorced their father shortly after Dylan was born and they had not had any contact with him since then. Early in our first session together I discovered that both boys were not only avid Chicago Blackhawk fans but, according to Catherine, "outstanding hockey players." I spent a lot of time finding out about the positions they played, what techniques and strategies they used to help them score goals, and who their favorite Blackhawk players were. Both Dylan's and Jaime's favorite all-time Blackhawk was Bobby Hull. The brothers had future aspirations of becoming pro hockey players. It was clear that I had engaged the boys around their interest and active involvement in the world of hockey. During my intersession break, I included hockey language in both the rationale for and the description of the therapeutic task. I shared with the family that it sounded like they were losing the game because the boys' *slap shots* were being directed at the wrong target and the *pucks* were missing the real *goal.* I also shared my concerns with the boys that they would continue to lose games (receive their mother's groundings, lose privileges, not be allowed to play in games), unless they started *scoring goals* with their mother by letting her be their cheerleader at home and at games. As an experiment, I left it up to each boy to pick one thing he could do over the next week to *score a goal* with his mother. Once a *goal* was *scored,* Catherine was to give the *hockey player* a high-five and a privilege of her choice. One week later, the mother reported that each boy had "scored two goals apiece" with her.

The last two important elements to consider when selecting and designing therapeutic tasks are family members' unique cooperative response patterns and the family's treatment goals. Once we determine in our relationship with each family member how he or she wants to cooperate in the change effort, we can carefully match our therapeutic tasks with where the family member is at in the cycle of change (de Shazer, 1985, 1988; Prochaska et al., 1994). Family members inevitably provide us with clues to how they want to cooperate with us. Our job as Sherlock Holmes-type detectives is to listen for and observe carefully clues from family members as to how they want to cooperate and change, particularly from how they respond to our questions, relate to us, and manage in-session family play or art therapy tasks. Finally, whatever therapeutic tasks we select or design have to be in line with the family's treatment goals. Once we have clearly elicited from family members what their ideal treatment outcome pictures will look like, tasks selected or designed should provide the *how* of empowering them to get there in the most concrete, manageable, and efficient way.

IDEA-GENERATING STRATEGIES
FOR CREATIVE PROBLEM SOLVING

As therapists, we can be as creative as we allow ourselves to be with any given client problem situation. The more ideas we generate, the greater the odds we will stumble upon a high-quality solution (Van Gundy, 1992). We need to be careful not to get locked into habitual ways of viewing particular types of client problems and rigid therapy model formulas for trying to solve them. The danger in being too wedded to one particular therapy model for problem solving is that it will rob us of the opportunity to test our own creative powers in coming up with a second, third, or fourth potential solution, which may be much more effective than a particular therapy model's first-choice intervention. The five idea-generating strategies that follow can tap our creative abilities and help generate high-quality solutions for challenging child presenting problems.

Mind Mapping for Solutions

Mind mapping was originally developed by educator and creativity expert Tony Buzan (1984, 1989) based on his years of research on note-taking skill development, learning, memory, and creative thinking with college students. In his research, Buzan found that the best note takers shared two unique characteristics: (1) They recorded key words used by the lecturer or the authors of the books the students were required to read; and (2) they kept their notes clear and easy to read. Writing down key words stimulates creative association and recall, making the gathered information rich (Buzan, 1984, 1989; Gelb, 1995). In a clinical situation, we want to listen carefully to the key or main words that family members use to describe the presenting problem and write them down as part of the mind map. For example, if a mother uses the words "bad attitude" to describe the cause of her son's behavior, we would want to write that down. Mind mapping works by creating a positive feedback loop between our brain and our notes. As an idea-generating tool, it trains us to organize our thoughts in a way that makes it easier to see the bigger picture and the details and to integrate logic and imagination. By capturing a tremendous amount of information on paper, mind mapping can help us to see the relationships, connections, and patterns of our ideas (Gelb, 1995).

The four steps to the mind-mapping procedure are as follows:

1. Draw a symbol or a picture in the center of the sheet of paper to represent the family's presenting problem.

2. Print family members' key words used to describe the problem.

3. Connect the family members' key words with lines radiating out from the symbol or the picture.

4. Use color coding or pictures to help produce greater associations; yellow can be used to highlight the most significant or key client words used to describe the problem, blue can be used to highlight the secondary most important key client words (Buzan, 1984; Gelb, 1995).

Because 80% of our brains is involved in visual processing at any given time (Ostrander, Schroeder, & Ostrander, 1994), we tend to learn faster and remember longer by using pictures of things. Therefore, pictures in mind mapping serve as "memory anchors" for key word associations and help us be more imaginative in our thinking (Gelb, 1995).

Besides simply mind mapping the problem alone, which in some cases generates useful solutions for the client's presenting problems (see Figure 4.1), I use mind maps in four other ways for creative problem solving. I map the opposite of a client's presenting problems. A map can be constructed of the words that family members use to describe their ideal treatment outcome pictures. Sometimes I think of a metaphor for the client's presenting problems and mind-map them. Finally, when stuck, I may pull out the dictionary and randomly pick a word to mind-map to see whether this triggers some useful ideas for solving the client's presenting problems (deBono, 1992). The following case example illustrates how mind mapping a problem can help generate potential solutions.

Fanny brought in for therapy her two sons, 6-year-old Albert and 8-year-old Harry, for "constantly arguing" with one another and not responding well to her "rules." Fanny reported that "the boys will not listen" to her unless she "yells" at them at the "top of her lungs." Both boys also voiced their upset feelings about the family's

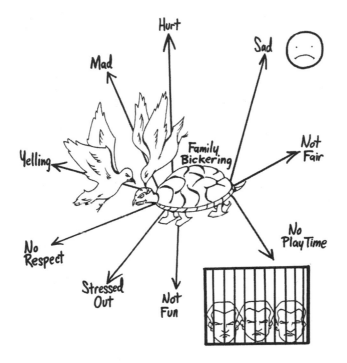

FIGURE 4.1. Mind map of family bickering problem.

bickering problem, particularly not liking their mother's "yelling" at them "all the time."

Fanny was a single parent; the boys' father disappeared when they were toddlers. Fanny was at her wits' end in trying to manage her sons' behaviors. She had taken all their toys away and prohibited them from going outside for a few weeks. It appeared that the more Fanny yelled and imposed lengthy punishments, the more out of control and oppositional the boys became. This was the destructive interactive dance the family was locked into.

I provided some parenting education for Fanny regarding the need for us to move away from yelling and inadvertently reinforcing the very behaviors she wanted to eliminate with her sons. She could not identify any past successes she had had resolving other behavioral problems with her boys. Together, we broke down Fanny's main problem concern area—the boys' oppositional behavior—into more solvable outcome terms: "not bickering with me" when asked to do things or follow her rules. When I attempted to externalize (White, 1995) the family bickering problem, I got strange looks from all family members as if they found this new construction of the problem to be bizarre. We also discussed the importance of Fanny having more time-outs away from the boys. As an experiment, I gave Fanny an observation task to keep track on a daily basis of what the boys were doing when they were not pushing her buttons. At the intersession break, I constructed a mind map of the family bickering problem (see Figure 4.1), which contributed to the boy's oppositional behavior.

To symbolize the problem, I drew a picture of a snapping turtle in the center of the page. I connected lines from the turtle to the key words family members used to describe the problem: "mad," "sad," "no respect," "stressed out," "not fun," "no play time," and so on. I drew pictures of two angry birds pecking on the turtle next to the word "mad," a face with a frown on it next to the word "sad," and three heads behind prison bars in a window next to the words "not fun" and "no play time." I then highlighted in yellow marker the words "mad," "not fun," and "no play time." After mind mapping, I came up with four ideas to present to the family: (1) Fanny should go out with a friend or on a date when she needed a break from the boys; (2) each boy could throw up a time-out hand signal with one another when conversations were escalating into possible arguments; (3) the boys, with their mother's permission, could go outside to play and take a break from being with the family; and (4) the boys could be put in charge of planning a fun family outing, as it had been more than a year since the family had gone out together. From this menu of intervention ideas, the family selected the first, third, and fourth tasks with which to experiment.

As this case example illustrates, mind mapping can offer therapists a quick and effective method for generating creative solutions. I ended up seeing Fanny and her family four times over a 6-month period. All family members reported changes in the bickering and oppositional problem areas by the second family session. Fanny discovered that once she stopped screaming and reinforcing negative behaviors with her boys, they became more cooperative and compliant with her rules and expectations. Family members found that having periodic time-out periods from one another and going on fun family outings contributed to everyone getting along better when together.

Imagine You Are the Problem

Gordon (1992), in his creative problem-solving research, found that the most important element in innovative problem solving was "making the familiar strange" because breakthroughs depend on "strange" new contexts by which to view a "familiar" problem. One way of making the familiar strange is for the therapist to imagine he or she is the client's problem. Empathically, the therapist identifies with the problem. For example, if I became a child's lying problem, I might ask myself the following questions:

"How do I think?"

"How do I feel?"

"What keeps me going in this family?"

"What am I scared of?"

"Why do I prey on this child?"

"What's funny or absurd about me?"

"What has to change in this family for me to go away?"

"What are the pros and cons of being this problem?"

Imagining ourselves as the problem not only can help us better understand the client's problem but can generate creative ideas for problem resolution. Jonas Salk, the polio vaccine pioneer, imagined himself as an immune system and contemplated how to fight the polio virus from that perspective (Gelb, 1995). The following case example illustrates how to use this idea-generating strategy in clinical practice.

> Simon was 10 years old and troubled by a chronic encopresis problem. His parents were both professors at a major university. The parents, particularly the father, expected Simon to excel academically in school. The father was constantly putting pressure on Simon to do his homework and to study. Simon's grades had dropped from straight A's to A's and B's. The frequency of Simon's soiling problem increased from four times a week to almost daily. No physical or medical problems were contributing to the soiling problem. Prior to being brought to me for therapy, Simon had seen several social workers and psychologists. The parents and Simon were very pessimistic.
>
> The miracle, coping, and pessimistic questions (Berg & Miller, 1992; de Shazer, 1988; Selekman, 1993) failed to produce any

exceptions. When meeting alone with Simon, he disclosed how mad he was at his father for putting so much pressure on him with school.

At my intersession break, I imagined that I was Simon's encopretic problem. In self-reflecting as the problem, I thought about how I was getting even with Simon's father by shitting on him and how absurd it was because it did not change him but just made Simon's situation worse. As encopresis, I was feeling mad and frustrated. I wondered whether, if I stopped preying on Simon, he could tell his father directly to back off a little with the school pressures. Simon had never confronted his father about this issue. Rather than giving this family a task, I decided in the editorial reflection to voice the above questions as encopresis. Suddenly, Simon took a risk with his dad and voiced his angry and frustrated feelings about the school issue. This proved to be newsworthy to the parents, particularly the father, and some useful dialogue followed between Simon and his father. In facilitating the dialogue, I got the father to agree to back off with the schoolwork pressures, providing Simon did the best he could in school. Also, we decided to reinstate father-and-son outings on Saturdays, which had stopped because Simon's grades declined. Simon and his parents were very pleased with the outcome of our meeting. The encopresis problem was completely resolved in six sessions. The father also committed to staying off Simon's back about school.

Attack the Problem from Different Angles

When feeling stuck with a case or unsure about which therapeutic tasks may be useful with a family's problem situation, it can be advantageous to attack the problem from many different angles. Sometimes I hop into my imaginary helicopter to gain an aerial view of myself and the family to help generate some new ideas. Wujec (1995) recommends looking at the problem situation as if it were "a statue to be examined from several points of view" (p. 64). Wes "Scoop" Nisker, a Buddhist and author of the book *Crazy Wisdom,* wrote the following about approaching problems from different angles:

> Crazy wisdom gets wise and crazy by gaining many perspectives: by changing points of view, getting into another place or a distant space and looking at things from there; by finding an odd angle, climbing high for an overview, seeing what is behind it all or underneath it

all, stepping outside or going inside. There are many ways of looking at things. (1990, p. 12)

The following case example demonstrates how stepping out of a family session in process can free the therapist to come up with some new ideas. An added bonus for the therapist is that abruptly leaving the session prior to taking his or her intersession break thus changing the therapy context, can help disrupt destructive family interactions.

Kit and Maggie, ages 6 and 7, respectively, were brought for therapy by their parents for "always fighting over every little thing." The parents reported that they "destroy" each other's toys and "kick and hit" one another. When asked about their attempted solutions, the parents started to blame one another in the session. The mother felt that her husband was "too strict." The father felt that his wife was "too lenient." While the parents were locking horns, both children started fighting over the toys they were playing with. As the father yelled at the children, their behavior escalated. I dismissed the children and met alone with the parents. Attempts to elicit from the parents an initial treatment goal proved to be futile, for the couple could not agree on anything. They began to blame one another for the children's behavioral problems. I decided to ask the miracle question (de Shazer, 1988) as a way to break up the blame–counterblame pattern of interaction. In the middle of the miracle inquiry, the couple began to lock horns again. I decided at this point to get up and check my mailbox as a way to do something dramatically different and to disrupt the couple's destructive interaction pattern. While at my mailbox, I came up with two potential therapeutic tasks that I thought might work for the couple. When I returned to my office, both partners began to laugh and the husband said, "You needed a break from us, right . . . huh! huh!" The parents seemed to have mellowed out in response to my improvisational move. I decided to present the two task ideas to the couple so they could choose which one they would like to try.

The first task option was for both partners to observe on a daily basis what the other does in relationship to the children that they like or think is good and to write those things down and bring the information in to our next session. They were not to compare notes until our next appointment. The second task option was the "structured family fighting task" (de Shazer, 1985; Selekman, 1993). The couple were instructed to get a kitchen timer and find a quiet room in the house to perform this task. The partners were to flip a coin and select heads or tails to determine who goes first. For 5 minutes the heads partner can argue with the other partner, who is patiently listening and making direct eye contact. Anything left over to complain about must be written down on a piece of paper and used for the next scheduled fighting session. Once both partners have had a turn, they are not allowed to fight again until the next scheduled fighting session time. The couple opted to try both tasks. They also began to take responsibility for their poor role modeling for their children. I provided support and encouragement to the couple and got them fired up to do the tasks.

I ended up seeing this family five more times. The parents returned to our second session reporting a wealth of changes. Both parents reported a lot of parenting qualities and behaviors that they appreciated about each other. After the first scheduled fighting session, they experienced difficulty in arguing with each other in session. The children's fighting behavior problem and sibling conflicts were resolved by our fourth family session.

Direct Analogies

Another useful idea-generating strategy is to think about what a particular family or problem situation reminds us of. Some of the families I have worked with have reminded me of a family on a TV show or in the movies. I once worked with a family that reminded me of the family in the movie *The Great Santini,* which starred Robert Duvall as a general who ran his family like the military unit. Over the years, I have worked with a number of Italian families that reminded me of Cher's family in the movie *Moonstruck.* Not only can analogies take the form of popular TV or movie celebrities, but family members or particular presenting problems can be compared to comic strip or book characters and animals, insects, and other aspects of nature. Many famous historical figures successfully used analogies to solve problems. Nobel Prize winners Crick and Watson compared DNA molecules to a spiral staircase, which helped them come up with their double helix theory of genetics. Physicist Niels Bohr thought of an atom as being like a miniature solar system (Prince, 1992).

I may use the direct analogy idea-generating strategy to help me get more playful with a family. For example, I think of a name of a new situational TV comedy show to call a particular family in my head.

Sometimes I think of a headline in a major newspaper that would best describe a particular family with which I am working.

> Rhonda, the mother, and Harold, the stepfather, brought in 10-year-old Stuart and 9-year-old Liza for therapy because they would not respond to Harold's limit setting and "tried deliberately to push his buttons." Rhonda's children were reportedly "pulling pranks" on Harold and sometimes "trying to hurt" him. Both Stuart and Liza were bitter about their physical and verbal mistreatment by their biological father. The parents had been divorced for 3 years. According to Rhonda, she was "battered" and "psychologically abused" by her "alcoholic" ex-husband as well. Because this was a war-torn family, I decided to give family members plenty of room to tell their painful past stories. While listening to Rhonda and Harold's present concerns about the children's pranks and their aggressive acts, an image flashed in my head that these children reminded me of Pugsley and Wednesday of the *Addams Family*. The family also seemed therapeutically ripe for externalizing the "anger" and "mistrust" problems that ran rampant in this family. All family members were being pushed around by these problems, including Harold. I decided to tap into the children's strong ability to be aggressive and mischievous in helping them and their parents defeat these problems that were haunting them from the past. Both children got very excited about drawing on paper the clever ways that they could defeat these problems. By the end of our first session together, Harold and Rhonda began viewing the children and the presenting problems in a new light.

Imagine the Problem Is Solved

When I am at a loss for ideas or feeling stuck in a family session, at my intersession break I pretend that the family's presenting problems were miraculously solved after they left my office. I allow my curiosity to run wild with the many possibilities now available to the family and to me since the problems were solved. Not only do I visualize what the changes will look like with the family, but I also watch myself doing things therapeutically differently with them that will be contributing to and maintaining the solution patterns. The following case example illustrates this idea-generating strategy in action.

Joshua, 8 years old, was brought for therapy by his parents for "low self-esteem" and "withdrawn" behavior and because he "isolated himself" from family members. The parents appeared to be very concerned and committed to helping Joshua. I asked the imaginary wand question to try to generate some possibilities and treatment goals and to better engage Joshua. Although the parents had no problem coming up with their ideal outcome pictures, Joshua had little to say. The parents also shared with me that Joshua was a "very shy child" and that it "takes awhile" for him "to trust new people." The parents' attempted solutions consisted of "not allowing him to isolate himself in his bedroom," "forcing Joshua to participate in social activities," and "making him go out to play with his friends." When the parents backed off in the past, Joshua tended to isolate himself in his bedroom or not to go outside after school. The parents could not think of anything that they were doing or had done in the past that helped Joshua be less withdrawn and more sociable. When I met alone with Joshua, I gave him plenty of space to talk and choose what play or art activity he would like to try. Joshua would not talk to me or invite me in on his play activity. I was feeling very stuck at this point in the session and took my intersession break.

I closed my eyes and imagined what Joshua and his family would look like when I reconvened with them and all of their problems were solved. I had this picture of the parents playing a game or drawing pictures with Joshua on the floor, then offering him choices of what game he would like to play in the session or asking him what team sports activity he would like to get involved in through their local recreational board. I saw Joshua smiling and happier now that he had more of a voice in his family. I saw myself in this session and in future sessions being more playful, asking less questions, and putting Joshua in charge of choosing a family art or play activity for his family.

When I reconvened the family, I found myself more relaxed and optimistic about change happening with this family. The parents welcomed the idea of giving Joshua more room to make choices. In future sessions, Joshua was put in charge of selecting the in-session family and art play activities. By our eighth family session, Joshua was not isolating himself anymore, was much more verbal, and appeared happier. The parents also discovered that Joshua responded well to their giving him the "responsibility ball" for making choices rather than forcing him to do things or deciding for him.

SOLUTION-FOCUSED THERAPY TASKS: OLD STANDARDS THAT WORK

The three Solution-Focused therapeutic tasks presented in this section are like old jazz standards that aficionados never get tired of listening to. A classic tune, whether played by a jazz great or a young new musician, will work for most listeners. The same is true for all three of the therapeutic tasks discussed here, which were developed by Steve de Shazer and his colleagues at the Brief Therapy Center in Milwaukee, Wisconsin. De Shazer and his colleagues have repeatedly demonstrated that these tasks are highly effective with a wide range of client presenting problems (de Shazer, 1988, 1994; Gingerich & de Shazer, 1991). Gingerich and de Shazer (1991) found, through their expert system computer program BRIEFER, that these tasks have a high probability of working when accurately matched with clients' unique cooperative response patterns. After describing each therapeutic task, I provide case examples.

Prediction Task

The Prediction task (de Shazer, 1988) is particularly useful with child cases in which the reported exceptions occur on a random basis and are not deliberate (i.e., the exceptions just happen out of the blue). I use the Prediction task to help increase the frequency of exceptions and assist family members in becoming more aware of what works.

> Rico, a 9-year-old Puerto Rican boy, was brought for therapy by his mother, Marcella, for "bad temper tantrums" which occurred on the average "four times per week." Marcella was unaware of what she or Rico was doing on the other 3 days of the week that made them "good days." The twosome typically fought over doing schoolwork, watching too much TV, and buying toys Rico wanted. Rico was very athletic and was a Michael Jordan basketball fan. I could tell he was a real competitor. I gave Marcella and Rico the Prediction task. Separately, the night before the next day, Rico and Marcella were to predict whether the next day would be a "good day" (no temper tantrums) and try to account for what made it a good day. I requested that they both play good detectives for me so we could figure out what works.

The family came back 1 week later and reported a number of changes. There were fewer power struggles, "only one temper tantrum" occurred, and Marcella was so pleased with Rico's changes that she bought him the "Nike Michael Jordan T-shirt he wanted." Marcella found that "yelling less" and "avoiding power struggles" seemed to prevent temper tantrums. Rico discovered that when he didn't give his mother a hard time "she yelled less" and they got along better.

Do Something Different Task

With child cases in which the parents' goal is not related to the reported exceptions, the parents' superresponsible behavior is contributing to the child's superirresponsible behavior, or the parents are stuck trying to win the power struggle battles with their child, I utilize the Do Something Different task (de Shazer, 1985). I explain to parents that their child has "got their number," he or she knows every move that they are going to make. After this short rationale for their need to be less predictable, the parents are given the following directive: "Between now and the next time we meet, I would like each of you to do something different, no matter how strange, weird, or off-the-wall what you do might seem" (de Shazer, 1985, p. 123).

> Kip, 10 years old, was brought for therapy by his mother for "constantly swearing," "talking" to her in a "disrespectful way," and "not doing his chores." Kip and Charlotte, the mother, were also having "daily arguments" about doing his homework. Charlotte did report that Kip was a "good student" and "can be a big help" to her "at times" around the house. Charlotte was at the "end of her rope" with Kip and was "seriously thinking about sending Kip to live with his father" out of state. I met alone with Charlotte and gave her the Do Something Different task (de Shazer, 1985) to perform as an experiment.

In 1 week's time, Charlotte came up with seven things that she did differently around Kip. One day she walked around the house all day with an ape Halloween mask that she found in a drawer. She bought a squirt gun and "squirted Kip" every time he would "swear at" or "talk back" to her. Once Charlotte changed her parental dance steps around Kip, he had to change his behavior to accommodate to his mother's changes. Charlotte became "less stressed out" and discovered that "parenting" could be "fun." We also successfully implemented the Compliment Box strategy.

Pretend the Miracle Happened

If the family is unable to identify any exceptions or the exceptions that have occurred are not newsworthy, I use the Pretend the Miracle Happened task (de Shazer, 1991). I meet alone with the child and have the child pick 2 days over the next week to pretend to engage in the parents' miracle behaviors to blow his or her parents' minds! I also ask children to watch carefully how their parents respond to them when the children are pretending.

> Tabitha, 9 years old, was brought in for therapy by her mother for what their "pediatrician" diagnosed as "school phobia." For 2 months, Tabitha had refused to go to school. No matter what her mother tried to do to get her to go to school, Tabitha would either "say she was sick" or "refuse to get out of bed." Despite the present behavioral difficulties, Tabitha had begun the school year by going to school without any problems. Other than Tabitha's willingness to attend school back then, neither the mother nor her daughter could identify what made this big exception possible. After asking the miracle question (de Shazer, 1988), Tabitha had little to say about her ideal miracle picture. Her mother, on the other hand, reported several miracle behaviors, such as "Tabitha would get up in the morning and go to school without any battles," she would have a "better attitude about school," they would be "getting along better," and she would "not hear any excuses about not going to school." I used scaling questions (de Shazer, 1988, 1991) to help establish a well-formed treatment goal with the mother. The mother's goal was for Tabitha to go to school at least 1 or 2 days over the next week. Although neither family member gave me any clues about how the school refusal problem developed, I did find out from Tabitha that she was upset with her mother because her mother had taken her "computer away" from her for the "past two months." I met alone with Tabitha to see if I could use the computer as a bargaining chip. Tabitha quickly warmed up to my proposal of trying to win back her computer for her provided she would be willing to try an experiment of mine. Tabitha was now on the edge of her seat. I asked her to pick 2 days over the next week to blow her mother's mind by pretending to engage in her mother's miracle behaviors. For the first time in the session, I felt that I had gained therapeutic leverage with Tabitha. She desperately wanted her computer back.

In 1 week's time, Tabitha went to school for an entire week! The mother was totally thrilled that Tabitha agreed to go back to school without any battles. I was able to negotiate with the mother to get Tabitha's computer back. A verbal contract was established between the mother and Tabitha that Tabitha would lose the computer again if she started to refuse to go to school again.

CONCLUSION

When selecting or constructing tasks for a family, it is important for therapists to have the family perform the same task in second and subsequent sessions if it continues to work for them. Therapists and clients get into trouble when they stop doing what is working. Any tasks selected or constructed for a family should fit with the family's problem definition; capitalize on their strengths, language, and beliefs; cooperate with the unique cooperative response patterns of family members; and be in line with their treatment goals. In this chapter, I have presented several different ways that therapists can generate creative ideas for effective problem solving and find fit with task selection and design. It is my hope that therapists will find the idea-generating strategies discussed in this chapter to be most useful for stimulating their creative juices and aiding in designing unique and original therapeutic tasks for their client families.

CHAPTER 5

Curious George Meets Dr. Seuss: Family Play and Art Therapy Strategies

The world of reality has its limits; the world of
imagination is boundless.
                            –JEAN-JACQUES ROUSSEAU

One day, after reading *Curious George Takes a Job* to Hanna, my 3-year-old daughter, I began to wonder what would happen if Curious George got lost and somehow stumbled into a Dr. Seuss story. Being an avid Dr. Seuss fan, I wondered how well Curious George would get along with Marco in *And to Think That I Saw It on Mulberry Street*, or with Horton the elephant in *Horton Hatches the Egg*, or the moose Thidwick in *Thidwick the Big-Hearted Moose*. Would Dr. Seuss try to rescue Curious George if he got lost in the Desert of Drize by providing him with a Crunk-Car or a Zumble-Zay? Finally, I wondered whether Dr. Seuss would want to try to teach Curious George a lesson about the dangers of being too curious. I came to the conclusion that Curious George would get along quite well with Marco, Horton, and Thidwick, that he would make it out of the Desert of Drize unscathed, and that, by the end of the story, Curious George would be quite a bit wiser about when to take risks and when not to.

Like Dr. Seuss, I want to coauthor stories with families that are filled with adventure, laughter, and surprises; stories that stimulate wonder and imagination. In each session, I want the family to learn something new about themselves that can make a difference in their thinking and doing. I want to break up any unhelpful beliefs held by the child and his or her family that keep them stuck and help them see that all they needed and wanted was already inside them. As Milton H. Erickson pointed out, "We know a lot more than we think we do; we have vast, untapped reservoirs of ability" (cited Ostrander et al., 1994, p. 178).

In this chapter, I present several family play and art therapy tasks that are Dr. Seuss-like in that they can successfully help family members step outside their familiar rational worlds and enter a world of imagination, where anything is possible. The unique needs of the family and what makes the most sense therapeutically dictate whether to select one or a combination of family play and art therapy tasks to implement in second and subsequent sessions. For example, for rigid families that have forgotten how to play together, the Family Mural, Imaginary Time Machine, or Invisible Family Inventions tasks can be most beneficial.

I conclude the chapter by discussing three highly effective visualization techniques that can be used with children.

MAJOR FAMILY PLAY AND ART THERAPY TASKS

In this section, I present seven major family play and art therapy tasks. I describe each family play and art therapy task and offer helpful guidelines about when and how to utilize them in the treatment process. Case examples help demonstrate the utility of each of these therapeutic tasks.

The Family Squiggle Wiggle Game

Winnicott (1971a) originally developed the Squiggle Wiggle Game as an effective therapeutic tool to assess the child's problem situation, his or her thought processes, and emotionally laden material about his or her family, as well as to help build rapport with the child in a fun and playful way. When working one on one with a child, the original Squiggle Wiggle format can be modified and used as an indirect method to introduce to the child new ideas or potential solutions for his or her presenting problems. These ideas can be embedded in the therapist's squiggle picture and story and reflected back to the child. The Family Squiggle Wiggle game is particularly useful with young children or children who have difficulty expressing their thoughts and feelings with family members.

When the identified child client is quite young or not very verbal, I invite him or her to select a family member to draw a squiggle on a sheet of paper and then ask the child to create a picture out of the squiggle and tell a story to the family and myself about the picture. The identified child client's picture and story can be quite newsworthy to the family; it can better help them understand what the child is going through and how the child views himself or herself and can reveal individual or family secrets or how the child views the family or their social world. Once the identified child client's picture and story are adequately discussed, he or she draws a squiggle and has the family create a picture and tell a story about it. Most families tend to create a picture and story that incorporate the identified child client in a positive way. Sometimes family members gain valuable insight from the identified child client's picture and story, or are so shocked by it that they request the opportunity to change the child's picture and the ending of the story to have a better outcome. The case example described next is a good illustration of this clinical situation.

> Luis, a 6-year-old Puerto Rican boy, was brought to the family session by his parents, who were very concerned about his "withdrawn" behavior, not socializing with "other children" in the neighborhood, "day dreaming in class," and looking "very sad" all the time. Luis's 14-year-old sister, Wanda, also accompanied the parents to this session. After multiple family moves, the family now lived in a gang-infested neighborhood, and intense feuding was going on between Luis's father, Carlos, and Carlos's cousin Ricardo. Recently, Luis had witnessed his father in a fistfight with Ricardo. The mother, Victoria, was on Prozac for her own "clinical depression." For the bulk of our first family session together, I had great difficulty engaging Luis. The imaginary magic wand question, trying to engage him in a board game, and using humor proved futile with Luis. However, I remembered that earlier in the session Victoria had said Luis liked to draw. So I decided to try the Squiggle Wiggle Game with him. I drew a squiggle on the construction paper, which not only elicited a smile from Luis but seemed to spark his curiosity. His parents and sister had their eyes fixed on Luis's paper. Suddenly, after Luis drew a picture of himself crossing the street about to be run down by a truck, Carlos voiced his concerns about wanting to save his son and asked Luis if he could draw a "stop sign" on the street and a "police crossing guard." Victoria and Wanda also got on the floor and asked Luis's permission to draw their additions as well. The mother drew an

"underground walkway" so that Luis would be able to "cross safely" to the other side of the street. Wanda drew a "police car with flashing lights" knifing in between Luis and the truck to save his life.

Family members were totally shocked by Luis's picture. They had no idea that he wanted to die. Although Luis remained very quiet, nonverbally he appeared to appreciate his family's concerns about him, which he indicated by smiling and showing interest in what family members had to say and what they were drawing. When the family returned 2 weeks later, the parents and Wanda reported a wealth of changes. Luis was socializing more with family members and peers, appeared to be in "happy spirits," and was much "more talkative." I was quite shocked by Luis's many changes as well. This was not the same boy I had seen 2 weeks earlier. The parents attributed Luis's changes to his expressing himself in our last session. Luis disclosed that he was "happy" now because his father and the cousin were "friends" again. I ended up seeing the family for one more session 6 weeks later to assess the family's progress; they reported no further problems.

Marshall McLuhan once said, "Art as radar acts as an 'early alarm system,' as it were, enabling us to discover social and psychic targets in lots of time to prepare to cope with them. Art, like games, is a translator of experience" (1964, p. 214). Through the use of the Family Squiggle Wiggle Game, Luis was offered a context in which to express his sad feelings about the chaos in his life and successfully rally his family around him for support. Like an "early alarm system," family members could graphically see in Luis's drawing his crying out for their help.

The Imaginary Feelings X-Ray Machine

For children who are not that verbal or have difficulty expressing their feelings, the Imaginary Feelings X-Ray Machine can be quite useful. The child and his or her family are told the following: "If I had an Imaginary Feelings X-Ray Machine that could show me what feelings you have inside, what would I see in the X-ray pictures?" I then have the identified child client lie on his or her back on some meat packing paper rolled out on the floor. The child can select a family member to draw an outline of his or her body on the paper. Once the contour of the child's body has been drawn, the child is to draw with magic markers or paint pictures within the lines of his or her feelings, as depicted in X rays taken of them. When the child is done, the X-ray results are processed with the family and the child. Other family members can perform the task as well. This task can be used in children's groups with similar results. It has been my clinical experience that children find this family art task to be fun and tend to become more aware of their own emotional world. Family members also tend to be surprised when they visually discover how the identified child client feels about himself and the family situation.

> Robbie, 9 years old, was brought for therapy by his mother, Phyllis, for "school behavior problems," "getting into fights" with peers, and breaking his mother's rules. Robbie's parents had been divorced for 3 years. The father, Conrad, was an "active alcoholic" and used to be verbally abusive toward Robbie and Phyllis. Conrad was inconsistent with visitations and Robbie was "very difficult to manage" for Phyllis when he returned from a weekend visit with his father. Phyllis's prime reason for bringing her son in for treatment was that she felt that he needed to "talk about his feelings about his alcoholic father." Apparently, Robbie always ran out of the room when Phyllis tried to get him to talk about his father. Phyllis called herself an ACOA (adult child of an alcoholic) and was actively involved in Al-Anon. Her father died from alcoholism. In the first session, I connected well with Phyllis and we worked on some parenting strategies. Robbie and I failed to click even after several attempts to get "in the door" with him.
>
> In our second family session, I decided to try the Imaginary Feelings X-Ray Machine task with Robbie, and he responded with excitement. Robbie's X-ray picture proved to be quite revealing. He drew a volcano erupting on the left side of his chest area. After drawing his heart, he put a padlock on it, so nobody could get inside. With the help of the Imaginary Feelings X-Ray Machine, Robbie was better able to talk about his anger toward his father (the erupting volcano) and how his father had repeatedly "hurt" him by forgetting promises to take him to the baseball game or to buy him things. The padlocked heart was symbolic of Robbie's unwillingness to allow himself to be hurt by his father anymore. Another important change was Robbie's seeking out his mother to talk about his "bad" feelings when upset at home or when thinking about his father. With the help of the Imaginary Feelings X-Ray Machine, we were able to better open up the lines of communication between Robbie and his mother.

The Family Portrait

Most art therapists use family drawings as an assessment tool for eliciting from children how they view themselves in the context of their families. Using family drawings, children can teach us about family interaction patterns, coalitions, conflicts, and how they view themselves in their families. DiLeo (1973) identified two common observations of family dynamics in children's family drawings: *omission of a family member* and *omission of self.* In the first family theme, the child may omit from the drawing a family member with whom he or she is in conflict, who he or she is rejecting, or who he or she feels rejected by. The second family theme is characterized by the child's placing himself or herself at the very end of a series of family members. Such children may view themselves as having low status in the family. It is even more significant when children place their younger sibling before them in the chronological sequencing of family members (DiLeo, 1973). Similar to the previously discussed family art therapy tasks, the family portrait can be used with younger children and children who are not very verbal and as a therapeutic pathway for challenging family patterns and beliefs. The following case illustrates the power of the child's family portrait drawing in challenging family patterns and for opening up space for possibilities.

> Jacob, 7 years old, was brought by his mother, Amanda, for counseling for his "low self-esteem," "spacing out in class," "ADD," and isolating himself in the family. Jacob's 6-year-old sister, Jeanette, was deemed a "gifted child" by her teacher. The father, a successful businessman, could not attend this initial family session due to his work schedule. Jacob was very shy and did not open up much to me. To get a better handle on how he viewed himself in his family, I invited Jacob to draw a family portrait. Amanda was totally blown away by Jacob's drawing. Not only did he put himself at the very end of all of the family members, but he also positioned himself slightly back behind the rest of the family. Unfortunately, Jacob did not have much to say about his drawing. In our next family session, the father was very concerned about Jacob's drawing. The father's presence in the session appeared to bring Jacob to life. He was better able to talk about not seeing his dad that much because of business trips and how he felt that "Jeanette always got her way." After sending the family to a neurologist for the "spacing out" problem, it was determined that Jacob had a seizure problem. Jacob's teacher had mistakenly labeled this problem as a symptom of ADD. Once Jacob was placed on the right medication and his father set aside more week-

end time for him, his symptoms both at home and at school rapidly stabilized.

The Imaginary Time Machine

The Imaginary Time Machine task can be used at any stage of treatment. It is particularly useful when a therapist is stuck with a case because it can propel the treatment system into possibility land. The therapist tells the family the following: "Suppose I had an Imaginary Time Machine sitting over here, and I asked each of you to enter it and take it wherever you wished to travel in time, where would you go?" "Who would you be with?" "What would you do there?" "What difference would that make in your life?" Family members can allow their imagination to run wild in terms of where they want to transport themselves or the family in time. When using this playful and fun family task with children and their families, I have been impressed with their tremendous creativity. Family members have come up with the following time traveling scenarios: one family transported its members back in time to a fun and marvelous family vacation; one child transported himself and the family into the year 2500 where they lived on a spaceship orbiting around Mars; an 11-year-old African American boy transported himself back to World War II to secure a Sherman Tank to bring back to the present to help defend himself against a neighborhood gang that had been hassling him on the streets; and an 8-year-old Mexican girl transported herself back to the neighborhood where her family used to live and she had lots of friends, unlike her present reality, where she had in the new suburban community in which she had no friends.

What is most powerful and effective with this therapeutic task is its ability to give families a vacation from their problems and help generate solutions for their presenting difficulties. Traveling into the past allows family members to remember past successes, such as useful coping and problem-solving strategies and fun things their families used to do to get along with one another. After going back to a place in history, a family member may want to bring back the creative ideas and wisdom he or she learned while with a famous personality of those times. By transporting oneself into the future, anything is possible because it has not happened yet. Osborn (1993) pointed out that "when we look forward to something we want to have come true, and we strongly believe that it will come true, we can often make ourselves make it come true" (p. 33). Two case examples demonstrate the effectiveness of this therapeutic task:

Kirby, 10 years old, was brought for therapy because of his "disruptive behavior" in class, "oppositional" behavior, and "lack of respect for authority." According to his mother, Sandra, Kirby was a "very bright" and "talented young man" who was "underachieving" in school. There was much conflict between Kirby and his stepfather, Herbert. Herbert and Sandra had been married for 2 years. Kirby's biological father, Sid, had not been in contact with him since the parental divorce, when Kirby was 5 years old. Present in the first family session were Kirby, Sandra, and Herbert. After getting absolutely nowhere with the miracle question (de Shazer, 1988), coping questions (Berg & Gallagher, 1991; Selekman, 1993), and the use of humor, I decided to improvise and try the Imaginary Time Machine task.

Kirby got excited about the task and wanted to go first. After entering the time machine, Kirby went back in time to join Sir Edmund Hillary and his team on their historical climb of Mt. Everest in 1953. Kirby had recently learned about Sir Edmund Hillary in class. Although Kirby was quite cold while traversing the mountain, he was thrilled about accomplishing the great human feat of being one of the first people ever to make it to the top of Mt. Everest. While describing this adventure to the family and me, Kirby appeared entranced by this experience, as if he were really there.

When processing the Mt. Everest experience with Kirby, he made it quite clear how "boring" he found his life, particularly his teacher. Not only did Kirby wish he could go to a more intellectually stimulating school, but he wished the family could go on an adventure vacation together. Sandra read into Kirby's Mt. Everest experience his "thirst" for a more "intellectually challenging education" and the need for "more variety" in his life. Herbert, an avid cyclist, came up with the idea of taking Kirby on a weekend cycling trip. Kirby appeared to warm up to this idea. We were able to get through the past conflicts Kirby and Herbert were having about the completion of chores. We also revisited the school situation in our third family session, which eventually led to Kirby's transfer to a "wonderful private school" program that Sandra had been trying to get him into.

The next case example involves a depressed 10-year-old girl who was underachieving in school and lived in a chaotic home environment. Her father had been incarcerated for armed robbery.

Melinda was brought for therapy by her mother for "failing three subjects in school," "looking depressed," and "testing" her mother's limits. Melinda's parents were divorced as a result of her father's "alcohol and drug abuse problems," "violent" behavior toward her mother, and "yelling" problem. Melinda really missed her father and had a tendency to defend him when her maternal uncle and cousins would "say bad things about him." In the first session, I had great difficulty engaging Melinda, particularly in eliciting from her what she would like to get out of family therapy. Her mother, Alice, did most of the talking and appeared to be overly concerned about Melinda's academic performance problem. My use of the miracle question (de Shazer, 1988) and humor failed to lighten up the atmosphere in the therapy room or create any possibilities with the family. After introducing the Imaginary Time Machine task to Melinda in our second family session, she came to life! Melinda transported herself back to the days of Pocahontas. Pocahontas took Melinda "through the woods" and taught her about nature and how to make clothing out of animal hides. Pocahontas and Melinda became "close friends." Melinda was in a total trance state while describing her special encounter with Pocahontas.

To further capitalize on their special relationship together, I had Melinda and Pocahontas hop into the imaginary time machine and ride it back to 1996. I explored with Melinda what advice Pocahontas would give her and her mother to help them get along better. According to Melinda, Pocahontas would tell her and her mother to "stop arguing" as much, for her mother to defend her when the uncle and cousins would put down her father, and for both of them to "listen better" to one another. When asked about how Pocahontas would be helpful to Melinda at school, Melinda pointed out how she would be "paying more attention" in class, "concentrating better" on her work, and "taking home and completing" her daily homework assignments.

With Pocahontas as my co-therapist, I was able to open the door for possibilities with this family. We were able to improve communications in Melinda's relationship with her mother, particularly by getting Alice to defend Melinda when the uncle and cousins would put down her father. Melinda also brought her failing grades up to a C.

Invisible Family Inventions

Similar to the Imaginary Time Machine task, the Invisible Family Inventions task stimulates creative problem-solving abilities with family members and invites them to play together, which may be a novel experience for families plagued by entrenched negative patterns of interactions and fixed beliefs about their problem situations. This task can be used at any stage of treatment. I begin the task by telling the family the following: "If you as a group were to invent something that could benefit other families just like you, what would that be?" I try to avoid giving the family any ideas, leaving the imagination process up to them. Once they achieve success with this task, family members discover that they can work together as a team without conflicts or problems, which proves to be a newsworthy experience for them.

Some examples of patented invisible family inventions, are a "chilling out" cylinder-shaped tank into which family members can go when they have an "attitude problem" or are ready to "blow" their "stack" with another family member; family jet packs to transport the kids around more quickly, thus freeing up one mother to run errands or do things for herself; and a special TV with a screen the family can walk through to join the cast of their favorite TV shows or to become a new character in video action-packed games.

> Samantha, a bright 10-year-old, was brought in by her mother for "constantly arguing about everything." Raquel, Samantha's 6-year-old sister, accompanied them to the session. Samantha's parents had recently divorced after a 1-year separation. Samantha was "refusing to do her chores" and was starting to associate with "troublemakers" in their neighborhood. Despite all the behavior problems, Samantha managed to get B grades in school. I had discovered earlier in the session that her favorite subject was science. As a way to lighten up the tension in the room and move the conversation away from complaints both the mother and Samantha had for one another, I presented the Invisible Family Invention task to the family. Samantha took a leadership role in trying to brainstorm ideas with her family. She came up with a most creative idea. She invented a "pill that families could take" when they are plagued by chronic "arguing" problems. According to Samantha, once ingested, family members are unable to "swear," "yell at," or "blame" each other. Instead of the negative responses, family members can only utter "compliments," "praise," and low-volume positive responses to one another. The positive effects of the pill were mostly contributed by the mother, with some help from Samantha. They both were in agreement that such a pill would "make families stronger" and probably would "make the world a better place to live" in.

By the end of our session, the atmosphere in the room had lightened up considerably. Samantha and her mother decided to take the invisible pill on a daily basis as an experiment, to see if it would help them "communicate better." Two weeks later, the family returned in better spirits, reporting that the pill had helped them "get along better." In closing our session, I suggested that they try to market their new pill and get the Food and Drug Administration to approve the pill for other families to help them with their problems.

The Invisible Family Invention task is wonderful in that it helps families generate their own unique solutions for their presenting problems by having them come up with creative ways for helping other families. Samantha's creative pill invention served as a pattern intervention strategy and a constant reminder for both Samantha and her mother that they could only interact with one another in a positive way, particularly under the influence of the pill. Interestingly enough, whenever Samantha and her mother were tempted to push each other's buttons, an image of the pill would flash before their eyes and prevent them from being negative with one another.

Child as Director of the New Family Drama

When working with families that have been chronically oppressed by their difficulties, in which the child appears to be locked into the family-scapegoat role or in which there is a lack of playfulness and family fun, I will do the following: I put the child in charge of one or more therapy sessions, to act as if he or she were the director of a TV drama or sitcom about his or her family. From behind a videocamera, the child directs family members how to behave and converse with one another. The therapist can play the role of the child or an absent family member. As the director, the child can be as creative as he or she likes with the themes, storylines, family role behaviors, and humorous elements of the new family drama/sitcom. The therapist and the family review the videotapes of each episode that the child directs and produces, and the child takes the lead in offering editorial comments.

The benefits of this family play therapy task are threefold. First and foremost, the child's competencies shine through when given a voice and empowered. Second, outmoded family beliefs about the child and unproductive family interactions are changed. Finally, family members become much more playful and spontaneous with one another, helping to liberate them from their oppressive problems.

The following case example illustrates how this family play therapy strategy can create possibilities with a stuck case.

Pedro, an 11-year-old Mexican boy, was brought into therapy for constantly testing his mother's limits, not doing his chores, and underachieving in school. His mother, Maria, was at her wits end with Pedro. She had a stressful managerial position with a company, and was tired of coming home from work and having to "yell at Pedro about everything." Her other child, Theresa, 10 years old, was an honors student at Pedro's school and "never misbehaved."

The first and second sessions proved to be highly unproductive in identifying a realistic and small treatment goal, as well as in trying to break up the blame–counterblame pattern of interaction between Maria, Theresa, and Pedro. When meeting alone with Pedro, I discovered that he felt blamed for everything and that his mother favored Theresa over him.

In my third family session, I decided to improvise and capitalize on one of Pedro's strengths and main interest areas, filmmaking. At school, Pedro was considered to be the most talented member of the school audio-visual crew. I showed Pedro how to use my videocamera and explained the director's task to the family. For the first time, the mother and Theresa began to respond to Pedro in a more positive way. While filming and directing his new TV show, he had me pretend that I was Pedro preparing dinner for his mother, with Theresa's assistance, in the kitchen. They made spaghetti and a salad for dinner. When Maria came through the front door, she was greeted at the door with hugs and kisses by the children and was escorted over to the nicely set dining room table for dinner. Throughout the filming of this first episode of the new family drama, there was much laughter, smiles, and comments from the mother like "How nice," "That was so sweet," and so forth.

Needless to say, this family session proved to be highly successful at disrupting the long-standing blame–counterblame pattern in the family and altering outmoded family beliefs about Pedro. I ended up seeing the family four more times and collaborated closely with concerned school personnel. Besides consolidating gains and amplifying changes, we implemented many of the creative ideas for improving family communications that Pedro had come up with while directing and producing the new family drama.

Stuffed Animal Team

With very young children, ages 2 to 5, I utilize their favorite stuffed animal friends as co-collaborators in the solution-construction process. As part of the engagement process with children, I explore with them who their favorite book, TV, and movie animal characters are. I then inquire whether the child has stuffed animal versions of these characters at home. Finally, I share with children that Winnie the Pooh, Barney, Clifford, Curious George, and their other favorite stuffed animal friends can be a big help to us while we are working together by helping to make them "happier," "less mad," "not scared" anymore, and so forth. Because most children are at the peak of their imagination and pretending abilities during the toddler and preschool years, typically they are quite excited about the idea of having their stuffed animal friends participate with them in therapy sessions.

I generally pursue this therapeutic strategy midway into the session after I have a clear understanding of the presenting problem and what the parent's goals are. I meet alone with the child and have the child introduce me to each of the stuffed animals, telling me what he or she likes best about each one. In a highly concrete way, I talk about the presenting problem and then inquire with the child what each of the stuffed animals would do to try to resolve his or her problem. I ask the following kinds of questions:

> "If Winnie the Pooh was sad, what would he do to make himself happy?"

> "If Curious George was scared, who would he go to for a hug?"

> "What would Clifford the red doggy tell you to do to make you happier?"

To the best of my ability, I also represent the voices of the celebrity stuffed animals and share with the child the various creative ideas and solutions each of the animals whispered in my ear. If the child wishes to be the voice of each of the stuffed animals, he or she can do that as well. Some children tend to have better imaginative abilities with this task than do others. Often, with the help of the stuffed animal team, the child can generate some creative problem-solving strategies and solutions. Before ending the family session, I have the child bring the stuffed animal team in to meet the parents and have him or her share with the family what creative problem-solving strategies and potential solutions the stuffed animal team came up with.

Rodney, a bright 4-year-old, was brought in for therapy by his parents for "trying to hurt" his baby sister, Lisa (9 months old) on several occasions. Ever since Lisa arrived in the family, Rodney had "mishandled" her in a "rough" way, "thrown things at her," and engaged in "attention-seeking" behaviors with his parents. The parents had tried everything from "time-outs" to "modeling" to teach Rodney how to handle Lisa in a "caring and gentle" manner, but he continued to "misbehave." The parents were feeling totally stuck and "frustrated." They could no longer leave Rodney alone with Lisa.

Throughout the first session, the parents were highly pessimistic. I normalized for the parents some of Rodney's attention-seeking behaviors as being a typical response to having to "share center stage with a new sibling." I further pointed out how the firstborn child often feels "dethroned" by the baby. The parents agreed and disclosed that they might have "spoiled Rodney," which did not help either.

Rodney was fairly quiet throughout the bulk of our first family session. Earlier in the session, I found out what Rodney's favorite toys were. Besides his Tonka trucks, his two most favorite stuffed animals were the Cat in the Hat and Tigger of Winnie the Pooh story fame. I suggested that Rodney bring the Cat in the Hat and Tigger into our second session to see whether they could help us out with the Lisa situation. In the second session, when meeting alone with Rodney, we discussed the problem and I asked him to talk to both the Cat in the Hat and Tigger to see what they would suggest to help him not hurt his sister. Rodney decided to pretend to talk for each one of them. When pretending to be Tigger, he hopped around the room and said, "Be funny for Lisa." I asked Rodney if Tigger thought he should "be a clown for Lisa to make her smile." Rodney thought it would be nice to be a clown for Lisa. As the voice for the Cat in the Hat, Rodney could also be a clown and sing songs for her. Rodney's favorite song was the "Hokey Pokey." With the help of the stuffed animal team, Rodney was able to generate two useful solutions which helped him get along better with his baby sister. The parents were very supportive of the ideas that Rodney and the stuffed animal team came up with.

I ended up seeing Rodney and his parents three times. Rodney greatly enjoyed being a clown and singer for Lisa, especially when she would smile and giggle. He also enjoyed all the positive attention he was getting from the parents by changing his behavior. His parents reported no further aggressive behavior toward Lisa.

EXTERNALIZING FAMILY PLAY AND ART THERAPY STRATEGIES

In this section, I present three family play and art therapy tasks to use with children and families when it makes sense therapeutically to externalize their presenting problems (Freeman & Lobovits, 1993; White, 1995; White & Epston, 1990). In challenging child cases in which the identified client is quite young or not very verbal, integrating art and play therapy methods with the Narrative Therapy approach (White & Epston, 1990) can be quite effective for empowering these children and their families to conquer their oppressive and chronic presenting problems in a fun way. Through the use of a variety of art media and family rituals, family members can tap into their creativity and playfulness to help create possibilities for even the most difficult and intractable presenting problems. Having the child go to combat with his or her family against the problem in the form of a family ritual or externalize the presenting problem in the form of a drawing on paper taps into the child's spirit of fun, which helps lead his or her family in the direction of change.

The Family Mural

Historically, art therapists have used the Family Mural task as a diagnostic tool to assess such family dynamics as communication problems, coalitions, parent–child conflicts, and so forth (Oster & Gould, 1987; Riley & Malchiodi, 1994; Sobol, 1982). Typically, the family is invited together to draw or paint a picture of themselves on a large sheet of paper. Sometimes the family is asked to illustrate themselves involved in an activity together (Kwiatkowska, 1978; Sobol, 1982). Although these two uses of the family mural can offer valuable insights about family roles, relationships, and perceptions of each other, outmoded family beliefs and entrenched patterns of interaction may remain intact. Therefore, I have found it to be more effective to use the Family Mural task as a visual therapeutic tool when engaging families in externalizing conversations. Through the use of externalizing questions (White, 1995; White & Epston, 1990), I first have the family co-construct the presenting problem into some objectified beast or thing, describing it in graphic detail (shape, color, demeanor, facial expression, etc.) and how it pushes all family members around. Sometimes the child and his or her family describe the problem in human form. Once there is some consensus about what the externalized problem looks like, I have the family draw a mural that depicts the various ways each family member interacts with the problem and how it gets the best of each of them. To help guide the family with the task, I might have them depict a recent scenario in which the problem was victorious over all of them. A second family mural can be drawn or painted that either depicts the various ways individual family members have achieved victories over the problem or illustrates in mural form a combat plan for defeating the problem. What is most remarkable with this family art therapy strategy is the resultant rapid and dramatic shift from the family viewing the identified client as the problem to the family group rallying around the child to prevent him or her from being further oppressed or victimized by the problem. The following case example illustrates the effectiveness of the Family Mural task with a difficult case.

> Peter, 9 years old, was brought for therapy by his mother, Marne, for chronic "stealing" and "lying." According to Marne, Peter had been "stealing money" from her since he was "5 years old." The lying behavior was a relatively "new problem." Peter had also stolen coins from his 10-year-old sister's piggy bank. Peter and his sister, Wendy, fought frequently, sometimes getting quite physical with one another, leading to one of the children getting hurt. Marne felt "totally frustrated" with Peter, for none of her "consequences" for Peter's acting-out behaviors worked. Prior to coming to see me, Marne had taken Peter to "five other therapists" and nothing had changed with his behavior. Seeing me was a "last-ditch effort" before trying to get Peter "placed in a group home." Peter was also feeling frustrated by his stealing and lying habits.
>
> I introduced the "habit" frame as part of the externalization process and as a new way for the family to view the stealing and lying problems. At a conference table, on which a large piece of tagboard was lying, I had the family brainstorm together how they would envision the stealing and lying habits if they were to draw them with magic markers on the tagboard. I also shared with the family that I wanted them to draw a recent scenario in which the stealing and lying habits were pushing all of them around. None of the family members could come up with an image for the lying

habit. Both the mother and Peter came up with the idea of drawing a bandit-looking man with a mask covering his eyes sneaking into Marne's and Wendy's bedrooms and stealing money from them. Each family member had already drawn him- or herself, so the mother's drawing of the stealing habit was a separate picture from Peter's drawing of himself, which was already drawn on the tagboard. Wendy drew herself yelling at Peter. Marne drew herself standing next to her children with her hands on her head, which was to indicate her frustration with the situation. We processed the family mural and all family members could clearly see how the stealing habit had a life of its own and was making them all feeling frustrated and mad, including Peter. Peter talked about how he felt like the stealing habit takes him over and brainwashes him to steal money from his mother and Wendy. By the end of our discussion about the family mural, both Wendy and Marne began to view and talk about the stealing habit as the real family villain. The family interactions changed as well. Family members stopped blaming Peter and offered their support instead. Wendy came up with the idea of hiding her piggy bank in a place where the "stealing habit will never find it." Marne thought this was a great idea for "tricking the stealing habit" and said that she would find a new hiding place for her money too.

I ended up seeing Peter and his family for four more sessions over a 6-month period. By our second family session, there had not been one stealing or lying incident or any fighting between Wendy and Peter. All family members talked about how they were not going to allow the stealing and lying habits to push them around anymore. The new family story that was evolving about Peter was that he was a "responsible young man." As the changes had occurred so rapidly with the family, I cautioned them to be on their toes because stealing and lying habits "do not die easily." The family saw this as a challenge to unite as a group and take measures to prevent themselves from becoming vulnerable prey to the habits. Wendy's idea about outsmarting the stealing habit by changing the location of her piggy bank proved successful. The mother also found this same solution useful in thwarting the stealing habit.

Drawing Out Problems

Another useful externalizing art therapy task is to have the child draw his or her problem on paper. It is crucial with the mechanics of this art task to give the child plenty of time to create an image or symbol to represent the oppressive problem that is pushing him or her around. To help guide the child with the art task, I ask the following questions:

"If you were to draw a picture of 'anger,' 'the attitude,' fears, etc., how would you make it look on paper?"

"What colors would it be?"

"Would it look mean, happy, sad, scary, etc.?"

These questions can be particularly helpful if the child is having trouble coming up with an image or symbol to represent the problem. Once the child has drawn his or her problem on paper, the therapist can invite the child to come up with a combat plan for defeating the problem on either the same sheet of paper or another sheet of paper. Children often feel empowered by this art therapy task; their problems are no longer controlling them from within their minds, and now they can control the problems after externalizing them on paper. I use this art therapy task with a child who is not very verbal or who tends to shut down when the whole family group is present. The parents can be called in to hear the child's story about his or her drawing and the child's combat plan. Typically, parents find it newsworthy to learn about how the child views the problem and its effects on him or her and the rest of the family. The parents can also be invited to help support the child's combat plan and offer any additional ideas to help the child defeat the problem. The parents can draw their ideas on the child's paper or on a separate sheet of paper.

> Raymond, 8 years old, was brought for therapy by his parents for "bad nightmares." According to Meredith, the mother, the nightmares had been pushing Raymond around for the past year. Apparently, Raymond would "wake up screaming in the middle of the night and run into" his parent's bedroom crying and seeking their comfort. The parents were totally perplexed by the nightmare problem. They could not identify any family crisis or changes, or anything else that could have caused the nightmare problem.
>
> When meeting with the whole family group, Raymond hardly talked and appeared very shy. His two sisters, 9-year-old April and 12-year-old Melanie, talked up a storm about themselves. My use of the imaginary wand question and humor failed to engage Raymond.

I decided to meet alone with Raymond and attempt to have him draw his nightmares. Using crayons, Raymond drew two different pictures of the "monsters" that were in his dreams. The first monster looked like a "ghost with big sharp teeth." The second monster was "big and hairy" and looked like a wolf man. We discussed what each of these monsters try to do to him when he is sleeping. The ghost monster would drape his sheetlike body over Raymond's head and try to "make it disappear." The other monster was more aggressive and would start "taking bites" out of him. I asked Raymond if he was getting scared talking about these monsters and he confidently answered, "No." I shared with him that I was getting scared hearing about these awful monsters. Raymond responded, "Don't be scared, they are only in my house."

Toward the end of the session, I had the parents come in to see the monster pictures. The parents could now understand why Raymond was having the bad nightmares. Knowing that the mother was talented with crafts, I suggested that she and Raymond make a "dream-catcher" together to place over Raymond's bed to prevent the evil monsters from pushing him around in the nighttime. I drew a picture on paper of what dream-catchers look like and shared with the family how Native Indian parents made dream-catchers to trap evil spirits that were trying to scare their children in the nighttime. By the end of our discussion, Raymond was much more animated and looking forward to making the dream-catcher with his mother.

I ended up seeing Raymond and his family three more times over a 4-month period. In our second session, Raymond was eager to show me the beautiful dream-catcher he and his mother had made together. Raymond also reported that he had not had one nightmare over the 2-week break period. After consolidating and amplifying the family changes, I predicted that the monsters might try to stage a surprise attack over the next-session interval period. To help safeguard against the potential sneak attack, I recommended that every morning Raymond and his mother carry the dream-catcher outside to let it air out after doing battle with the monsters the night before. I pointed out that monsters cannot survive outside the house and the smell of fresh air and the sunlight on the dream-catcher is lethal to these monsters. I further added that often the monsters disappear for good after doing this ritual one time.

The Habit Control Ritual

Once the child's presenting problem has been externalized, the Habit Control Ritual (Durrant & Coles, 1991; Selekman, 1993) can be used to empower the family to liberate themselves from the problem's reign over them. After externalizing the problem, I have the family keep track on a daily basis of the various things each family member does to achieve victories or to stand up to the problem and not allow it to push them around. At the same time, I want family members to keep track of the various ways they accept invitations from the problem to be pushed around by it or to lock horns with one another. I recommend to families that they keep a daily record of both their victories and the problems on a large piece of tagboard. Finally, I encourage families to work out together to be fit to defeat the problem.

In the session, I encourage the parents to serve as supportive coaches to the child when they see him or her accepting invitations from the problem to get into trouble. For example, a parent could say to her son, "It looks like the Temper is trying to make you not do your homework ... are we going to let it take away your TV time tonight or are we going to get the homework done?" I have the parents be their own coaches for their relationship as well, particularly when the problem is trying to make them argue with one another about how to manage the child's behavior. A father might say to his wife, "Why are we allowing the Temper to divide us again?" I also encourage families to meet as a group after dinner to evaluate how well they are doing at achieving victories over the problem and where they need to tighten up to be less vulnerable prey for the problem.

> Seven-year-old Sidney was brought for therapy by his parents for "severe temper tantrums," fighting with peers, and "attention-deficit/hyperactivity disorder" (ADHD). Sidney was adopted at the age of 1 by the Petersons. They had no other children. Ever since he had been adopted, the parents had described him as being "difficult" and a "behavior problem." The mother described him as being like the Looney Toon cartoon character the Tasmanian Devil. Apparently, when Sidney had temper tantrums, he would "leave a pathway of destruction from room to room." "Plates, pencils, books," and other projectiles would typically end up being "thrown into walls" and sometimes at the parents when Sidney had "bad temper tantrums." The parents had "tried everything under the sun" in the way of consequences, but nothing had worked. The

pediatrician had placed Sidney on Ritalin, which did seem to help him perform and behave better at school.

I decided to externalize the temper tantrum problem into "the Temper." After mapping the influence the problem had over Sidney, his parents, and the day-care instructor, it was clear that they all had been victimized by the Temper. Sidney did "not like the battles" with his parents and he wanted his family to be "happy." The parents disclosed that they had been "arguing a lot more lately" with one another. When I asked unique account questions (White, 1995), not one family member could identify anything he or she was doing that helped achieve victories over the Temper. In fact, the parents reported that more than half the time the Temper was victorious over them. I gave the family the Habit Control task as a way to help them become more aware of what they were doing daily not to allow the Temper to push them around, as well as to keep track of how the Temper got the best of them. We discussed the importance of physical training as a family and the parents' supportive coaching of Sidney to avoid accepting invitations from the Temper; I suggested they work together as a team to achieve victories over the Temper. Like a football coach before the big game, I got the family fired up to do team battle with the Temper.

Three weeks later, the family returned and reported a wealth of changes: 70% of the time they were victorious over the Temper, Sidney's behavior greatly improved at home and at the day-care center after school, and the parents were "arguing less." Sidney found that "forgetting" about the Temper worked for him at home and at the day-care center. However, a new Temper had invaded this family: "The Homework Temper" was now pushing them around.

The Homework Temper was not only sabotaging Sidney when he started to do his homework, but it was making Sidney and his mother lock horns. We brainstormed possible strategies that could help us defeat the Homework Temper. The parents decided that the father would monitor the homework situation and the mother would "back off." Also, Sidney decided to experiment with the "forgetting about the Temper" strategy that had worked so well for him.

At the end of the session, I had the family put their hands in the center to get them fired up to defeat the Homework Temper. Five weeks later, the family came back reporting that "88% of the time that the Temper was out of here!" Sidney was "doing his homework without any battles" and reported improvement in all areas of his life. Sidney and his father were also spending more quality time together. Mutually we decided to stop therapy because of the wealth of changes and the family's desire to test the waters on their own.

What was most remarkable about Sidney and his family was the way they worked so well as a team to quickly defeat both the Temper and the Homework Temper. Based on the family members' descriptions of the temper tantrums and their effects on them individually and collectively, the family seemed ripe for externalizing the problem (White & Epston, 1990). I had begun therapy by using a fairly pure Solution-Focused approach; however, the exceptions elicited by the miracle and coping questions (de Shazer, 1988; Berg & Gallagher, 1991) were not newsworthy to the parents because they did not fit with the dominant story that Sidney was the problem. Once the temper tantrums were externalized, the new construction or frame for viewing the problem proved to be quite acceptable to the family's beliefs about it. Sidney was also tired of being pushed around by the Tempers and the resulting "battles" that followed with his parents. Sidney was most impressive in spearheading the family's crusade and subsequent victories over the oppressive Tempers. He successfully helped his family trailblaze a "happier" lifestyle.

CREATIVE VISUALIZATION

During creative visualization, individual's use imagination to create what they want in their life. According to Parnes (1992), the "Visionizer," when pursuing his or her dream, "proceeds from examining 'what is' to exploring 'what *might* be,' to judging 'what *ought to* be,' to assessing 'what *can presently* be,' to deciding 'what *I will commit to do now*,' to action that becomes a new 'what *is*'" (p. 3). Visualization pioneer Wenger (1985) and Wenger and Poe (1996) stress the importance of describing "the dickens out of" the images when visualizing. Buzan (1989) has found in his research that people are more likely to attend to and remember something if it moves, is colorful, imaginative, exaggerated, and absurd. Bonny and Savary (1973) and Gordon and Poze (1981) have provided some empirical support for the importance of describing images fully in great detail in their imagery research. This mental process tends to synthesize the analytical powers of the left brain with the imaginative powers of the right brain (Parnes, 1992).

Ostrander et al. (1994) contend that if individuals imagine something vividly enough and with their heart bring their senses and emotions into play, their deep mind cannot know the difference between the imagined event and an actual one. The more of themselves they engage in the imagining process, the stronger the desired effect will be.

Two studies with children who experience learning difficulties have empirically demonstrated the efficacy of visualization techniques in improving their academic performance abilities. In the first study, Dr. Robert Hartley, of the University of London, took a group of children growing up in poverty who did poorly academically and as an experiment gave them the following directive: "Think of someone you know who is very clever," he told the children. "Now, be an actor. Close your eyes and imagine you are that very clever person and do the picture-making test the way he or she would." The children were successfully able to imagine they were clever and became clever. Their test scores rose considerably. Imagining they were someone else, in this case someone bright and clever, became a shortcut to expertise for them (Ostrander et al., 1994, pp. 149–150).

Rosella Wallace, an educational psychologist, used the Head of the Careful Observer technique with children to help improve their sense of self-awareness, articulation, and writing. Wallace had the children in her study imagine fitting a head of a careful observer over their own heads. She asked them questions to get them to describe aloud, with their eyes closed, this special observer:

"How does he act?"

"How does he approach objects, people, events?"

"Make him part of your imaginary world."

The children in her study found that they became superversions of themselves, using the observer's eyes, senses, and mind to perceive scenes as richly and vividly as the careful observer does. As Wallace put it best, "It's virtual reality without the equipment" (quoted in Ostrander et al., 1994, p. 155).

Some of the most famous people in history were great visualizers. Einstein once said, "Imagination is more important than knowledge." He attributed his scientific acumen and genius to what he called "vague play" with signs, images, and other elements, both visual and muscular (cited in Wenger & Poe, 1996). This "combinatory play," he wrote, "seems to be the essential feature in productive thought" (cited in Dilts, 1994, p. 48). One day Einstein visualized what would later become his famous theory of relativity simply by wondering what it would be like to run beside a light beam at the speed of light (Dilts, 1994; Wenger & Poe, 1996).

Other famous visualizers were Michelangelo and World War II hero General George Patton. Michelangelo imagined his sculptures as living beings, awaiting only his hammer and chisel to free them. He would also get ideas for new artworks by looking at the shapes of cracks in building walls. General Patton imagined that he was reincarnated from famous military generals of the past. He would apply many of these ancient generals' warfare strategies and tactics in modern-day combat (Ostrander et al., 1994; Wenger & Poe, 1996).

Children make excellent visualizers for a number of reasons. Young children in particular like to pretend, have a keener sense for wonder, and are highly open to suggestion. Children have very sensitive and thin-boundaried brains, which makes them unusually sensitive to people, forces, and external stimuli in their environments (Ostrander et al., 1994; Wenger & Poe, 1996). "Children's imaginations roam freely because they are not constrained by adult rules of thinking" (Wujec, 1995, p. 20). Their use of approximate thinking and undying curiosity provides them with a world of enchantment and possibilities.

In this section, I present three different ways I utilize creative visualization techniques with children. The case examples illustrate these techniques in action.

Imagine Yourself As . . .

For children who experience learning difficulties and behavioral problems, one highly effective visualization technique to help empower them to resolve their difficulties is to imagine becoming someone they greatly admire (Ostrander et al., 1994) (e.g., a famous person in history, a close friend they respect, or a TV, movie, or music world celebrity). Once the child has been able to access a crystal-clear image of the person he or she will become for a designated period of time, I have the child apply all his or her senses while visualizing. I ask the child to describe out loud, in present tense, with his or her eyes closed, the following:

"Where is the conversation taking place?"

"How is he or she dressed?"

"What is his or her facial expression?"

"What do you see him or her doing?"

"How does his or her voice sound?"

"What is he or she telling you?"

"What do his or her clothes feel like?"

The next step is to have the child access an image of him- or herself merging with the ideal other and becoming the other. Again, I have the child close his or her eyes and visualize him- or herself shaking hands with the ideal admired other and watching the latter disappear while the child becomes that person. Often, when the child becomes that admired ideal other in the session, the therapist can observe shifts in his or her voice, posture, and confidence level.

Before applying the Imagine Yourself As . . . visualization strategy to the child's presenting problem, I have the child practice becoming his or her selected ideal other a few times a day for a week, with the rationale that "the better you get at acting as if, the more easily you will become the person you want to be." After 1 week of solid practice, I have the child show me how quickly he or she can become the ideal other while visualizing. I then have the child see him- or herself as the ideal other, taking constructive steps to resolve his or her presenting problem. For example, one child I worked with averaged C grades on quizzes and at times was disruptive in class. During our session he "became the smartest kid in his class." The next day he went to school and not only secured A grades on two class quizzes but behaved well for the whole day. His teacher called his mother to share her amazement at how well he had performed on the quizzes and gave the child kudos for his behavior.

The following case also demonstrates the Imagine Yourself As . . . visualization technique.

LaTisha, a 10-year-old African American girl, was brought for therapy because of her "fears" of having to "talk or sing in front of others." According to the parents, LaTisha always got "panicky in class and at church" when she would have to give a talk or "perform with the children's chorus." Sometimes LaTisha would get so nervous that she would "start to cry or run off the stage" at church when performing. The parents were totally perplexed by LaTisha's fears, which began when she was 8 years old, for, to their knowledge, nothing had happened that could have caused this problem. LaTisha could not explain why she was having this problem either.

Out of respect for cultural differences, I explored with the family how they felt about working with a white therapist. The parents appreciated my asking them about this and acknowledged that they did not have a problem with it. I asked them if they had been praying hard for LaTisha to help her conquer the fear problem. Her mother in particular was praying daily for LaTisha. I got the parents' permission to meet alone with LaTisha to try the Imagine Yourself As . . . visualization strategy.

Because LaTisha loved the arts and was a very visual person in general, I was confident that this technique would work. LaTisha selected the pop music star Whitney Houston as her admired ideal other. LaTisha proved to be an excellent visualizer; she had no difficulty accessing a clear image of seeing herself become Whitney Houston. I had her practice becoming Whitney Houston daily for a week.

When the family returned for our second session, the parents reported that LaTisha seemed "more self-confident." LaTisha appeared more relaxed to me and happily reported that she found the visualization technique "helpful." However, the real challenge for LaTisha was 2 weeks away. She had to sing in a choral concert at another church in front of a large crowd. I had LaTisha continue to visualize herself daily performing as Whitney Houston, giving a great performance in the upcoming choral concert. As she had been to this church before and had a clear image of what it looked like, it was fairly easy for her to transport herself to that church and to see herself being a singing success.

Before I saw the family for our third session, I received a phone call from LaTisha's parents. According to the parents, LaTisha did an "outstanding job" and they were "so proud of her" performance in the choral chorus. Apparently, she had "held her head up confidently," singing throughout the whole concert. I complimented LaTisha on the phone and told her I too was very proud of her. We mutually agreed to get together in 1 month as there were no more signs of fears either at school or at church and things were going so well. Our third session ended up being our last session.

Visualization as a Cognitive Management Technique

Visualization techniques can be quite effective at disrupting the unhelpful thought patterns that are driving the symptoms of depressed and anxious children. The visuals can take many forms, such as having children visualize the problem as an icicle in their hand, a giant Karate chop hand chopping at the "bad" thoughts, or a stop light turning red. As part of the visualization process, I may access some of the children's other senses, such as seeing themselves listen to their favorite song being played at a high volume when they think negatively or are anxious. These visualization strategies are particularly useful when the parents have changed and are doing things differently around the child but the child is still symptomatic or plagued by intrusive negative thoughts.

Visualizing Movies of Success

Another way I use creative visualization with a child is to have him or her visually capture a past achievement or personal triumph when performing at school, in the arts, or in a sports event and use this internal movie as a road map for success in the presenting problem area. It is most important to have children engage all their senses in the visualization process and for them to describe for the therapist what they see, hear, feel, touch, and taste. Children can practice daily a few times a day accessing their visualization of success. The following case example illustrates the efficacy of the visualization of success technique with a challenging case.

> Levon, a 10-year-old African American boy, was brought for therapy by his mother, Ayeisha, due to "acting out in school," "problems with authority," an "attitude problem," and "not follow-ing" Ayeisha's "rules." Ayeisha was a single parent; Levon's biologi-cal father had "walked out" on her. She had two other children, LaTonya and Heather, who were at home being watched by Ayeisha's adult sister. Levon had not seen his father since he was 2 years old. Although Ayeisha described Levon as being a "talented athlete," she was quite upset with his "poor performance in school" and "lack of respect" for her and her rules.
>
> Earlier in the session, I checked out with Ayeisha and Levon how they felt working with a white therapist. Neither Ayeisha nor Levon reported any concerns about our racial differences. I di-vided the session up and spent some individual session time with both Ayeisha and Levon. Ayeisha was very pessimistic about the likelihood of Levon's ever changing. We agreed to work on some new parenting strategies together and I gave her an observation

task as an experiment. I had her keep track of anything she was doing daily to keep the situation with Levon from getting worse, even if it helped only a little bit. Levon was a little more challenging to engage than his mother. He was somewhat guarded with me in the earlier part of the session. I joined best with Levon when I had him talk about how he became the most valuable player for his football team 2 years in a row.

Levon had been playing on his public football league team for the past 3 years. He had led the league 2 years in a row in scoring the most touchdowns. He proudly shared with me that he had "scored 20 touchdowns" to cap off his most successful year as a running back. I asked him what his formula for success was, and he replied: "Stay low ... keep your legs moving ... spin when you get hit." I shared with him that "I thought I was listening to Walter Payton," the former Bears running back star. Levon laughed and shared with me that he liked "Walter Payton a lot!"

At this point, I decided to have Levon close his eyes and take me on a visual journey back in time to his best football game ever. He described for me a fairly recent game in which he had scored "three touchdowns" and had "gained 150 yards" on the ground. His graphic detail of this game literally put me right on the sidelines, watching him perform with excellence. Levon was animated, he could taste the sweat coming down his face, he could hear the crowd, and he saw clearly the corner of the end zone toward which he was running to score a touchdown. While heading for his third touchdown he broke three tackles. It was quite clear that Levon greatly enjoyed this visual trip back in time.

Using football metaphors, we talked about various ways he could "score touchdowns" both in school and at home with his mother. Levon admitted that he was tired of "fumbling" in school (getting poor grades) and that he needed to "stay low" and focus on his reading more. On the homefront, I suggested that he work on "spinning off" of his mother's "nagging" him and keeping his "legs and feet moving" toward getting his chores done. Finally, I prescribed for him to practice his visualization of his best game on a daily basis. I also asked him to notice how his teacher and mother respond differently to him when he is breaking tackles and scoring touchdowns with them.

By our next session, Levon had made considerable progress. Levon found that the visualization of his best game greatly helped him perform and behave better at home and at school. Ayeisha was very pleased with Levon's progress as well. The observation task helped her discover that not nagging or yelling at Levon seemed to help them get along better. We had two follow-up sessions to further consolidate gains and treatment was completed.

INTERPRETATION: A CAUTIONARY NOTE

When utilizing family art therapy tasks, it is crucial that the therapist be careful not to present his or her reflections about family members' art products as final explanations or truths carved in stone. Gestalt art therapist Janie Rhyne cautions therapists about avoiding what she calls "either/or dragon thinking," which leads to "putting clients into diagnostic boxes." She recommends the following when therapists become stuck in this way of thinking:

> The either/or dragon is a robot construction; he can be dismantled and reduced to powerlessness if we, person to person, can accept all of us as being in different places on the road of discovery and recognize that we can all learn some new directions from each other. (Rhyne, 1996, p. 29)

Tinnin (1990) suggests, when interpreting clients' art products, that "the therapist must be careful when converting a message from pictures into words to avoid unintentional distortion by his or her own verbal censorship" (p. 9). Typically, I invite family members to reflect on their own art products first and offer my own interpretations or reflections after each member's "voice" has been heard. My reflections are usually presented as "crazy ideas that just popped into my head" or with qualifiers of uncertainty, such as "I wonder if . . . " or "Could it be . . . ?"

The therapeutic power in family art therapy tasks is that the art representations of the family or self within the family provide an opportunity for family members to look at their problem situation "once removed." The family art task offers families a new lens for observing their situation and themselves as if they were outside their family system. Processing their art products with family members, increases the likelihood for them to find new themes and new histories, create an alternate view of their problem, and invent a new reality (Riley & Malchiodi, 1994).

CONCLUSION

In this chapter, I presented several family play and art therapy tasks and creative visualization techniques that can be utilized with a wide range of children's presenting problems. All these therapeutic tasks and techniques can be used at any stage of treatment. Most of the family play and art therapy tasks not only address the child's individual issues but produce changes throughout the family as well. Therapists will find in general that using the various tasks and techniques discussed in this chapter livens up their therapy sessions and makes their clinical work with families more enjoyable.

CHAPTER 6

Guidelines for Optimizing Therapeutic Cooperation in Second and Subsequent Sessions

I don't lead musicians, man. They lead me. I listen to
them and learn what they do best.
                                                    –Miles Davis

In second and subsequent sessions we typically observe four different
therapist–family member cooperative response patterns: *better, mixed
opinion, same,* and *worse* (Selekman, 1993). How well family members
manage and find the assigned therapeutic tasks dictates what the
therapist should continue to do or do differently in future sessions with
a particular family. As mentioned in Chapter 2, therapists need to
carefully match their questions and tasks with the unique cooperative
response patterns (de Shazer, 1985, 1991) and stage of change (Prochaska et al., 1994) of each family member. It is important to remember
that family members do want relief from their oppressive problem
situations, no matter how pessimistic or skeptical family members
appear. Therefore, carefully listening to and observing family members'
verbal and nonverbal responses to the assigned tasks provide us with
important clues to how they want to change. With children, the
therapist needs to assess whether the best way to cooperate with them
and promote change is through the use of in-session family play and
art therapy tasks, out-of-session therapeutic tasks, or a combination of
both. Some children tend to do their best therapeutic work either when
engaged in a board game of their choice or when participating in a

fun and playful in-session family task that taps their imaginative powers and ability to dramatize their family stories.

In this chapter, I provide guidelines for how to optimize therapeutic cooperation, amplify and consolidate family members' therapeutic gains, assess assigned task effectiveness, and constructively manage family member slips or setbacks with each of the therapist–family member cooperative response pattern groups. I also discuss how to empower highly pessimistic families, which are indicative of the *worse* family group.

THE BETTER GROUP

The *better* group often returns for a second or subsequent session looking different and reporting a wealth of changes in their problem situation. In general, it is most advantageous to begin the session with confidence and optimism and ask the family, "So, what's better?" Each reported family member exception pattern (new ways of feeling, viewing, and doing) needs to be carefully amplified and consolidated. The therapist should highlight differences by making distinctions with family members about old unhelpful patterns of behavior and outmoded beliefs and their new exception patterns of behavior and different ways of viewing themselves and their problem situations. Consolidating questions (de Shazer, 1994; de Shazer & White, 1996; Selekman, 1993; White, 1995) can effectively amplify the family's new solution patterns and make them more newsworthy on the meaning level for family members. Following are some examples of consolidating questions:

"How did you do that?!"

"How did you manage to take that big step?!"

"How did you come up with such a great idea?"

"What did you tell yourself that helped you to do that?"

"What else did you tell yourself?"

"What will you have to continue to do to get that to happen more often?"

"Is that different for your son to do that?!"

"Let's say we get together in a month, what further changes will you tell me you made?"

"Since you have made such great strides, have you gotten any new ideas about yourself as a parent that you would want others to know?"

"How will I know that you're confident enough for us to stop?"

"Do you have any new ideas about how you view yourself as a person now as opposed to when we first started working together?"

"What would you have to do to go backwards?"

"How will I know when things are better enough with your situation?"

"On a scale from 1 to 10, 10 being better enough, what number would you rate your situation today?"

"Let's say this was our last counseling session together; what fun things will you be doing during this time?"

"How will you celebrate your victory over the problem?"

"Who will you invite to your victory party?"

"What will you say in your victory speeches?"

After adequately consolidating family gains, the therapist should assess with family members whether they feel they successfully achieved their initial treatment goals, how they found the assigned tasks, and if or when they would want to come in for a future check-up session. The family members should be in the driver's seat in terms of determining how long they wish to remain in treatment and the frequency of appointments.

If there have been a number of family changes between sessions, it is most beneficial to give the family a vacation from therapy as a vote of confidence. By giving families longer time intervals between visits, we are giving them the empowering message that they have the tools and the strengths to make it on their own. While on vacation from therapy, the ripple effect triggered by the changes they achieved in treatment will be free to reverberate throughout the family system and other social systems with which the family interfaces.

Finally, if family members indicate that they found the therapeutic tasks assigned to them to be most helpful in generating out-of-session changes, the therapist should have them do more of what's working until they are confident enough to stop doing the tasks. In the editorial reflection, I prescribe that the family continue to use the same tasks and share with them the following rationale for doing so: "If it ain't broke, don't fix it." Families and therapists get into trouble when they stop doing what is working for them, which leads them to feel as if they are back to square one when they experience a minor setback.

THE MIXED OPINION GROUP

When families return for their second and subsequent sessions armed with concerns about their failure to make more headway in the goal area, or when other concerns arise, I normalize their concerns and share with them that change is a funny thing, that it often appears as "three steps forward and two steps back" (de Shazer, 1985). Before addressing family members' concerns, I first try to amplify, cheerlead, and consolidate the gains they have already made in treatment. I also point out to families that we are going for small changes here, which can eventually lead to bigger changes. If these interviewing strategies appear to be acceptable to family members based on their nonverbal and verbal feedback, I further empower the family by amplifying their changes and utilize a future focus through presuppositional and con-solidating questions (O'Hanlon & Weiner-Davis, 1989; Selekman, 1993). For example, I may ask a family: "Let's say we were to get together in four weeks, what further changes will you make happen by our next session?" The therapist can expand the possibilities with family members' visualizations of future success and explore with them where they will rate themselves on the scale in terms of goal attainment at this future time.

If some family members still have concerns, I shift gears and ask conversational questions (Andersen, 1991; Anderson & Goolishian, 1988a, 1988b) to give them ample space for storytelling, which may include ventilating emotionally laden material. The use of coping sequence questions (Berg & Gallagher, 1991; Selekman, 1993) also helps to create possibilities for more pessimistic or cautious family members. These questions are particularly useful with "yes, but ... " clients. Some examples of coping sequence questions are:

> "I'm curious, how come things are not worse with your situation?"
>
> "What steps have you taken to prevent things from getting worse?"
>
> "What else seems to help things from getting worse?"
>
> "How has that made a difference?"

It is also most advantageous for therapists to go back to basics with *mixed opinion* families by asking themselves the following questions:

"Do we have a customer here?"

"Is the treatment goal still too monolithic?"

"Are we working on the "right" client problem?"

"What tasks might better fit family members unique cooperative response patterns?"

"As a better way to cooperate with family members, should I offer them a menu of therapeutic tasks to choose from?"

"Do I know what the parents "key question" is about the problem?"

"Does the problem appear to occur on a random basis?"

Guidelines for Task Design and Selection for the Mixed Opinion Group

1. If one or both parents continue to be superresponsible around the child and/or participate in frustrating and unhelpful power struggles with him or her, prescribe the Do Something Different task (de Shazer, 1985).

2. If the problem/symptoms appear to be occurring on a random basis, prescribe the Prediction task (de Shazer, 1988).

3. If one or both parents undercut or put down the other parent's attempts to discipline or manage the children in the family, prescribe an observation task. For 1 week, have each parent observe what parental behaviors the other parent engages in with the children that he or she likes or approves of and write them down on paper. They are not allowed to compare notes until the next scheduled family session.

4. If the previously assigned task(s) from the first or subsequent session were partially helpful, or one or more family members disliked the task(s) assigned, the therapist should explore with them any ideas about how these task(s) can be modified or changed to their liking. The therapist can also brainstorm ways to simplify or improve the task(s).

5. The Secret Surprise task (de Shazer, 1985), which is a playful task for helping to generate more exceptions; it can challenge the parents' problem-saturated beliefs about the identified child client. Parents are often pleasantly surprised by the good deeds or nice things the child does to shock them in a positive way in 1 week's time.

6. If still stuck, use the idea-generating strategies described in Chapter 4.

Case Example

Isaac's mother, Mildred, spent the majority of our first family interview complaining about her overweight son's "overeating," "living off of junk food," and "refusing to stick with any sports activities" for which she would sign him up. Isaac's father, Sidney, had died from a heart attack and had been quite obese as well. Mildred's catastrophic fear was that unless she took steps now to help Isaac with his weight problem, he would eventually die from a heart attack like his father. When I met alone with Isaac, I found out that his mother was constantly nagging him about what he ate and pushing him to participate in athletics at school and through their local recreation board. Isaac reported that his mother's behaviors contributed to his feeling more anxious, powerless, and hopeless about being able to lose weight. When Isaac experienced these feelings he disclosed that he would "pig out" and eat foods that he knew were bad for him. Isaac could not identify any exceptions to this problem pattern. To assist Isaac with combating unpleasant emotional states and self-defeating thoughts, I taught him visualization techniques and how to decatastrophize (Seligman, 1995) his negative thoughts. I also prescribed that Isaac pretend to engage in his mother's miracle behaviors over the next week and observe how she responded to him when he was pretending (de Shazer, 1991). I gave Mildred the Do Something Different task (de Shazer, 1985) as an experiment to help disrupt her superresponsible pattern of interaction with Isaac.

One week later the family came back with mixed opinions about their progress. The transcription of the beginning of our second session illustrates how to address this therapeutic situation.

THERAPIST: So, what's better?!!

MILDRED: Not much . . . I mean yesterday he ate a whole bag of cookies!

ISAAC: Yesterday was a bad day for me, but I had a much better week!

THERAPIST: What steps did you take to make it a better week?

ISAAC: I ate fruit a few times over the week for dessert, instead of cookies or doughnuts.

THERAPIST: Wow! Is that a new thing for you to do?

ISAAC: Yeah, I think Mom would tell you that I rarely eat fruit or vegetables.

THERAPIST: Is that true, Mildred?

MILDRED: Yes, I was surprised by that, but . . .

THERAPIST: Isaac, did you eat some vegetables as well this past week?

ISAAC: I ate salad twice.

THERAPIST: Really? Is that new for Isaac to eat vegetables like salad?

MILDRED: Yes (*smiling*), I almost fell out of my chair when I saw him eat two large portions of salad.

THERAPIST: Isaac, have you gotten any new ideas about yourself in terms of eating better over this past week?

ISAAC: Yeah, I think I'm doing better with my eating and feel happier.

MILDRED: Certainly, I'm encouraged by his progress, especially his starting to eat a little better, but we still have days like yesterday and . . .

THERAPIST: I appreciate your cautiousness, this difficulty has been going on for a long time. I'm curious though, did you observe any other moments or days before yesterday where Isaac was showing you signs of progress?

MILDRED: Yes, in fact two days ago he agreed to sign up for Little League.

THERAPIST: Wow! How did you get him to do that?

MILDRED: The funny thing about that was that I didn't force it on him like I usually do. I just left the flyer on the dining room table. Interestingly enough, he approached me with a desire to play this year.

THERAPIST: Really? How did you come up with that clever idea to leave the flyer on the dining room table?

MILDRED: I don't know, I guess I am too pushy with him and need to give him more space to make decisions.

THERAPIST: Is he a good baseball player?

MILDRED: Yeah, when he used to play a few years ago he was a great slugger. Isaac has a good arm.

THERAPIST: Isaac, were you surprised when your mom gave you space to choose whether or not you wanted to play Little League?

ISAAC: Yeah, usually she tries to force me to do things.

THERAPIST: Besides letting you decide whether or not to sign up for Little League, did you see your mom do anything else differently that you liked over the past week?

ISAAC: Yeah, she didn't nag me as much.

THERAPIST: Were you doing anything else differently that helped your mom nag less?

ISAAC: I've been asking her to go with me on bike rides and to take me to the YWCA to swim.

THERAPIST: Wow! This young man's on a real health kick crusade! There's no stopping Isaac now! He's on a roll! That's worth a high-five! (*Both Mildred and Isaac smile.*)

As readers can clearly see, we made a complete U-turn from Mildred's initial pessimism to spending the majority of the session highlighting important changes that occurred in 1 week's time. Cheerleading was used to help reinforce and amplify family members' important behavioral changes and new ways of viewing themselves and their situation. Because both Mildred and Isaac were heading in the right direction for improving their situation, it made no sense to offer them any new tasks with which to experiment.

THE SAME GROUP

With the *same* group, some or all of the family members will be anxious to tell the therapist that nothing has changed with their problem-saturated situation. However, it is still helpful to explore with individual family members whether there have been any periods during which they experienced any slight improvement with their problem situation. Any reported exception patterns of behavior can be used as potential building blocks for solution construction, particularly if increasing the frequency of these useful problem-solving and coping strategies can empower the family to resolve their presenting problem.

If family members continue to be negative and cannot identify any exceptions occurring between visits, I shift gears and utilize coping sequence questions (Berg & Gallagher, 1991; Selekman, 1993). This may produce some important exception material on which we can capitalize that was not reported earlier in the session. Similar to the process with the mixed opinion group, the therapist should go back to basics and revisit with the family the following:

"Are we working on the "real" or the "right" problem?"

"Does the problem need to be renegotiated into more solvable terms?"

"Does the goal need to be renegotiated into more solvable terms or does the family want to establish a new goal area to focus on?"

"Do we have a customer participating in our sessions or do we need to further assess who the customer is in the client system?"

"Are there any new helping professionals involved with the case with whom the family thinks you need to collaborate?"

When further assessing customership, I may ask the identified client or other family members the following scaling question: "On a scale from one to ten, ten being most concerned about you, what numbers would you give absent family members or significant others?" A high number on the scale indicates that we need to expand the treatment system and engage these absent family members and significant others to aid us in the problem-solving effort. When new helping professionals get involved with the family's case, I get consent forms signed so I can begin collaborating with these helpers to try to develop cooperative working relationships with them. Conversational questions (Andersen, 1991; Anderson & Goolishian, 1988a, 1988b) can also be used to address family members' concerns.

Guidelines for Task Design and Selection for the *Same* Group

1. If the Do Something Different task has not been tried and it seems appropriate, prescribe it as an experiment for the parents, particularly if the parents are stuck engaging in "more of the same" attempted solutions (Watzlawick et al., 1974) to manage the child's misbehavior.

2. Track the problem-maintaining sequences of interaction and use pattern intervention (O'Hanlon, 1987) strategies, such as adding something new to the context in which the problem occurs, subtracting one element from the problem pattern, exaggerating the problem/symptom pattern, and so on. In Chapter 8, I present other pattern intervention strategies that can be utilized with parents.

3. If the family describes the problem as continuing to be oppressive and out of control or appearing to have a life of its own, I externalize the problem (White, 1995; White & Epston, 1990) and

design a ritual such as the Habit Control Ritual (Durrant & Coles, 1991; Selekman, 1993) to help empower the family to conquer the presenting problem.

4. When the parents have made some changes but the child is still symptomatic or not very verbal and the parents still have concerns, it may be worthwhile to implement the family play and art tasks, cognitive skills training, and creative visualization techniques.

5. If still stuck, use the idea-generating strategies described in Chapter 4.

Case Example

Stella brought her 7-year-old son, Horace, for therapy because he walked around "angry all of the time," had "temper flare-ups," and "hit" the neighborhood children with whom he played. The first session with this family was characterized by Stella's complaining about Horace's difficult behaviors and Horace's refusal to let me in the door to engage him. Not only did Horace refuse to answer my questions, but he would not play a board game or draw any pictures when I tried to involve him and his mother in a family art task. At the end of the session, I offered Stella an observation task to help me better understand what was working during the times Horace was not having difficulties.

One week later, Stella came back for our second session with a frustrated look on her face and quite pessimistic. She could not report one exception to Horace's problem behavior. To better match her pessimism, I asked, "How come you have not thrown in the towel with counseling? What keeps you trying?" Stella responded, "I'm hoping this behavior will pass ... I don't know ... maybe it's me ... I worry a lot?" I decided to track the problem-maintaining sequence of interaction between Stella and Horace. It was clear that Stella was stuck nagging and being too overprotective with Horace, which often led to Horace's temper flare-ups and his taking out his anger on a peer or destroying one of his toys. I offered Stella the Do Something Different task (de Shazer, 1985) as an experiment to try over the next week. When I met alone with Horace, he continued to treat me like I had the plague.

When the family returned for their third session, I did not recognize them. Smiles were plastered on both Stella's and Horace's faces. Apparently, Horace was in "good spirits" most of the week. There had been no temper flare-ups and no fights with kids.

When I inquired what Stella was doing that produced this miraculous outcome, she disclosed that she decided to stop nagging and "infantalizing" Horace. Stella observed that when she discontinued these two problem-maintaining behaviors, Horace's behavior greatly improved. I prescribed that Stella continue to do more of what was working.

I ended up seeing Stella and Horace two more times to consolidate gains. The biggest surprise for me in this session and the final two was that Horace initiated checkers games with me!

THE WORSE GROUP

Families that fit into the *worse* group category are often very pessimistic. Some of these families have experienced multiple treatment failures and have a tremendous dislike for therapists. Others have been plagued by multiple crises and problems that have been oppressing them for many years. Therapists typically run into a brick wall with such families when they tend to be too optimistic, do not provide the family with enough space to tell their problem-saturated stories, and fail to cooperate with their feelings of hopelessness and despair. Therefore, it is important to begin therapy sessions with pessimistic families by asking open-ended conversational questions (Andersen, 1995; Anderson & Goolishian, 1988a, 1988b) and operating from a position of "not knowing." To gain access to their beliefs about why their problems exist, and to make sure I have a good handle on what they view as the "real" problem, not what I or other therapists have thought is "the problem" that keeps them stuck. I want to give family members ample space to share their problem-saturated stories about negative past experiences with therapists. It is also quite useful to shift gears and cooperate with the family's pessimism and ask such pessimistic questions (Berg & Miller, 1992; Selekman, 1993) as the following:

"What keeps you going with this situation?"

"How come you have not thrown in the towel already?"

"What do you suppose is the smallest thing you could do that might make a slight difference?"

"And what could other family members do?"

"How could you get that to happen a little bit now?"

"Can you think of anything you used to do with your son or daughter in the past that seemed to be helpful, that we might want to test out now?"

It is also quite helpful to place families that are therapy veterans in the expert position and have them serve as consultants on how to best conduct therapy with them. I ask them the following questions:

"You have seen a lot of therapists before me, what did they miss with your situation?"

"What were some of the things these therapists did with you that you disliked the most?"

"In what ways can I be more helpful to you as a therapist?"

"In your minds, if you had the most perfect therapist to work with, what would he or she be like?"

"What would he or she ask you about or do with you that you would find most helpful?"

"If I were to work with another family just like yours, what advice would you give me to help them out?"

"If there was one question that you think is most critical for me to hear from you so I can best help you out, what would that question be?"

I have found it most helpful to have crisis-prone, pessimistic families predict what their next crisis is going to be; I elicit the details about who will be involved, where it will happen, and what effect it will have on family members. This therapeutic strategy can successfully disrupt their long-standing family crisis-prone pattern, especially if the therapist offers tools for effectively managing the future crisis situation. Also, while brainstorming collaboratively with the family about past successes, we may stumble on problem-solving or coping strategies that once worked and can be utilized as effective tools for achieving future successes. As with the *same* family cooperative response group, it is also important to go back to the basics with the *worse* group in terms of revisiting customership, the initial treatment goal, and problem clarification. Active collaboration with involved helping professionals is also critical.

Guidelines for Task Design and Selection for the Worse Group

1. Utilize pattern intervention (O'Hanlon, 1987) strategies to disrupt the family dance that appears to fuel the identified child's symptoms/problems.

2. Externalize the problem as a viable therapeutic option with highly pessimistic, war-torn families that describe their problems as chronic and oppressive in nature.

3. Use the idea-generating strategies described in Chapter 4 to design new therapeutic tasks that can aid in the change effort.

4. Use cognitive skills training, visualization techniques, or the family play and art therapy strategies discussed in Chapter 5 if the child's symptoms are not stabilizing.

5. If working solo, recruit a colleague or a few staff members to serve as a reflecting team (Andersen, 1991, 1995). Team members can offer you and the family some fresh, helpful new ideas for viewing the family's problem situation. The team is free to reflect on key family themes and the unspeakable, such as family secrets that may be driving the identified child's symptoms/problems.

Case Examples

Three case examples demonstrate my work with highly pessimistic multiproblem families. In all three of the cases, I felt a sense of stuckness early in treatment, as well as therapeutic paralysis in response to the parents' hopelessness and despair and the children's chronic and intractable symptoms.

> Lance, 5 years old, was brought in for therapy at the preschool teacher's request for "severe impulse control problems," "ADHD," "soiling," "bedwetting," and "low self-esteem problems" related to his "severe speech handicap." The parents, both recovering alcoholics, observed a major decline in Lance's behavior after the sudden and tragic death of his younger brother, Tony, following Tony's heart surgery.
>
> Tony had been born with multiple birth defects, including a heart valve problem. Initially, his open heart surgery appeared to go as well as possible. But Tony died in his bed 8 hours after returning home from the hospital. This was a terrible tragedy for everyone in this family. Both parents experienced bouts with

depression. Until the time I began seeing Lance and his family, he had engaged in a daily ritual of "searching through the house for" his deceased brother and "calling out his name."

For the bulk of our session, Lance could not sit still; he crawled under tables and my desk, and I could barely understand what he was saying because of his severe speech problem. One thing I did discover in my first encounter with Lance was that he enjoyed drawing. I made a mental note of this strength. The parents were very pessimistic about Lance's ever being able to get over the loss of his brother. Of all Lance's presenting problems, the parents considered the "real" problem to be whether he would ever "get over the loss of Tony." They were not concerned about Lance's other problems because they believed the "unresolved loss issue" was at the root of them.

I gave the parents ample space to talk about this issue. However, I was at a loss for coming up with potential solutions, particularly with getting a child this young to understand the abstract concept of death and to mourn this loss. Besides offering some parenting skills, normalizing Lance's regressive behaviors, and drawing with him, I had no idea where I was going with this family until our third session together.

Lance, with a little help from his mother, had put together a number of drawings of Tony and himself in book form. Once Lance created the book, his behavioral difficulties spontaneously began to improve. He stopped the ritual of searching throughout the house for Tony and calling out his name. It was as if Lance had naturally externalized his thoughts and feelings about missing Tony onto paper. He and his mother had found their own high-quality unique solution to the loss issue by creating a book about Tony.

I ended up seeing Lance and his parents seven more times over a year. An important part of the treatment process was actively collaborating with Lance's teacher. The teacher was quite burned out; she had "four other boys" in her class who "were major behavior problems." It was not until the time of our eighth family session that the teacher noticed that Lance had changed dramatically. The parents wanted to keep Lance in treatment over the school year as a result of pressure from the teacher and her superiors to keep him in therapy because of the pathology-laden psychological evaluation results that identified Lance as exhibiting ADHD. Lance was never placed on Ritalin. By our last session together, Lance was symptom-free, speaking more clearly, and sporting a sunny, happy face. As a reward for being a "big boy who was taking big steps," I gave Lance one of my favorite Nerf balls. The mother also took a picture of Lance hugging me as a way for him always to remember me, a similar strategy to that of creating a "Tony Memory Book." This was clearly a highly resilient and resourceful family. What I found most interesting about this case was that throughout the course of therapy, I discovered the power of "not doing." By giving family members plenty of space to tell their painful stories, they not only provided me with what they perceived as the real problem but generated their own unique solution, which was far better than anything I could have ever possibly come up with.

The next case example concerned a 10-year-old girl, Audrey, who had been described in past treatment summaries and psychological evaluations as "deeply depressed," "a hopeless case," "a damaged child," "ADHD," "behavior-disordered," and "severely learning disabled." Audrey had had four inpatient psychiatric admissions for "clinical depression" and was chronically "tearing up her clothes." Audrey had had a total of 12 outpatient therapy experiences. Her father had been psychiatrically hospitalized for "clinical depression" and had had several unsuccessful and "bad therapy" experiences. Her biological mother used to beat Audrey until she was reported to child protective services; at that point, Audrey went to live with her stepmother, Emily, and father, Jim. Audrey had one biological sister, Theresa, who was 17. Emily and Jim had four children together ranging in ages from 15 months to 8 years old.

In our first session together, only Emily and Audrey showed up. Although Emily appeared very committed to trying to help Audrey, she was highly pessimistic that Audrey would "ever change." Audrey was now having "difficulties getting along with" peers at her therapeutic day school, was still "destroying her clothes with her hands," and was stealing from her older sister, Theresa. Audrey was tall for her age and very fidgety and squirmy in her chair. She appeared to be extremely nervous and had little to say to me.

I decided to meet alone with Audrey to see if I could join with her over a checkers game. It was interesting to note that Audrey went out of her way to help me beat her in the game. Audrey did, however, disclose that she wished she had a closer relationship with her father, who was never around. I met alone with Emily to clarify what she perceived as the "real" or main problem, which turned out to be Audrey's "destroying her clothes with her hands." According to Emily, this was proving to be an "expensive bad habit" for her and Jim.

As I had discovered that Audrey "loved art" earlier in the session, I recommended that the mother buy some clay and find a quiet place in the house for Audrey to use her hands daily to make sculptures. Emily thought this was a novel idea and said she would implement this strategy immediately. In exploring past successes, I discovered that "going for long walks with Audrey" after dinner seemed to be helpful in curtailing some of her mischief-making behaviors. The mother had to stop these walks because of other parenting responsibilities. Jim "did very little" to assist her "with the kids."

After four sessions with Emily and Audrey, we successfully resolved the tearing up clothes problem. I also got a look at some of Audrey's "best" animal sculptures, which were quite good. Another important change occurred in the context of our checkers matches, Audrey was showing signs of wanting to win the games, no longer setting herself up to lose. She also appeared to be happier and more self-confident. Emily was very pleased with Audrey's progress both at home and at school. In fact, the special school that Audrey attended wanted to gradually start mainstreaming her back into a regular school in her district because of her "academic and behavioral progress."

I ended up seeing Emily, Audrey, and some of the other children eight more times over a 2-year period. I actively collaborated with Audrey's school throughout the 2-year period we worked together. Another big change was that Audrey beat me in checkers three times! Audrey also excelled in her classes in the regular school.

Throughout the course of therapy, I oscillated between feeling pessimistic and being hopeful that Audrey would change. My therapeutic optimism greatly increased once we resolved the tearing up clothes problem.

Mary, a highly depressed Kenyan woman, sought therapy for feeling like a "failure as a parent," wanting help for learning how to "better manage" her "difficult" and chronically oppositional 6-year-old daughter, Tomika, and having difficulties coping with her marital separation of 3 months. Another major stressor for Mary was the separation from her older daughter, Keisha, who was living with Mary's mother in Kenya. Mary did not have a green card so she could not freely leave and return to the United States after visiting her daughter. She had not seen Keisha for 5 years and felt "very guilty" about "abandoning" her.

When Mary first came to see me, she was severely depressed and had fleeting thoughts of wanting to kill herself. She was also presenting with a wide range of vegetative symptoms. Although Mary did not have a suicide plan, I made sure that she had some semblance of a support system. Mary and Tomika had been living with her "caring" and "supportive brother" Walter for the past 3 months after Mary separated from her abusive husband, Winston, who was also Kenyan. According to Mary, Winston used to "yell at" her all the time and found it "unacceptable" for her to "work." Whenever Mary challenged Winston, he would "scream at" her or "slap" her. As another way of exercising his power and control over Mary, Winston would not try to help her get a green card or brainstorm ways to secure a "visa for Keisha to come visit" them. Winston used to call Mary a whore because Keisha was a product of an out-of-wedlock relationship. Culturally, Winston was a tradi-tional African man. He believed strongly that Mary should adopt a subordinate position to him in regard to all decision making.

After securing a secretarial position for a small company, Mary and Tomika moved out and went to live with Walter. Throughout the session, I provided Mary with plenty of support, empathy, and room to tell her painful story. She spent a lot of time complaining about Tomika's oppositional behavior. Mary was also quite pessimistic about "ever being able to see Keisha again" and having the ability to change Tomika's behavior. Mary had been yelling a lot at Tomika, which seemed to make the situation worse. I gave Mary an observation task of keeping track on a daily basis of any encouraging steps on Tomika's behalf and anything she was doing to promote these prosocial behaviors. I also hooked Mary up with a psychiatrist to see whether an antidepressant medication was necessary. By our second session together, Mary had observed that her daughter was being less oppositional. However, Mary still felt quite hopeless about the future. In exploring her feelings of hopelessness, Mary disclosed that she went back and forth with the idea of "moving back to Kenya" so she could be "reunited with Keisha." Mary also "felt like a prisoner" in her marriage because of her strong religious beliefs about divorce being a "sinful act."

Tomika accompanied Mary to our second session. She ap-peared to be a very loving child who worried about her mother.

Tomika disclosed that she "missed not playing games" with her mother like they used to. I decided to have Tomika and Mary make a family mural drawing of how they wanted the family situation to look. Both Tomika and Mary seemed to have a lot of fun making the family mural together. Tomika drew her mother holding hands with her with a smile on her mother's face. She also added a big bright sun and colorful houses. Neither Mary nor Tomika added Winston to the picture. When asked about this, Tomika said she was "scared of" her dad and that he had done "bad things" to her mother. Mary disclosed that a strong part of her wanted to "start a new life" with Tomika either in the United States or back in Kenya.

I ended up seeing Mary and Tomika six more times. Mary was placed on Zoloft, which successfully stabilized her vegetative symptoms. By our last session, Mary had decided to leave Winston permanently. Tomika was no longer oppositional and the two of them were getting along much better. Mary had been saving up her money to get her own apartment. She had gotten a raise at her job. Finally, Mary had discovered that playing and drawing with Tomika tended to promote Tomika's prosocial behavior.

SOLUTION ENHANCEMENT: CONSTRUCTIVE STRATEGIES FOR MANAGING FAMILY SLIPS AND SETBACKS

Many families, while on vacation from therapy, experience some slippage backwards in the goal area or with their progress. Initially, family members may think that they are back to square one when this happens. Rather than perpetuating this unhelpful way of perceiving a slip or setback, I like to normalize such occurrences as being quite common and a critical part of the change process, and I share with the family the following:

> "We could not have made headway if we did not have a slip or setback."

> "When families change, it is similar to getting the hiccups, they come and then they pass."

> "Having a slip provides us with the opportunity for comeback practice" (Tomm & White, 1987).

After normalizing with families the inevitability of slips while they continue to change, I explore with them the steps they have already taken to get back on track prior to coming back for a tune-up session following the slip or setback.

When the family still feels derailed by their recent slip or setback, we brainstorm steps that they can take to get back on track. I inquire about past successes prior to the slip or setback. Here I ask specifically what the parents and other family members were doing that worked prior to the slip or setback. I may have family members gaze into my trusty imaginary crystal ball to visually capture the future steps they will be taking to stay on track.

CONCLUSION

In this chapter I presented several guidelines for optimizing therapist–family member cooperation and promoting change with families in second and subsequent sessions. It is important to remember that each session is a unique experience; therefore, how family members present themselves in second and subsequent sessions will guide the therapist in terms of deciding what type of question to ask or what type of therapeutic task to design or select. Thus, every therapeutic move the therapist makes in any given session needs to be purposive and to fit with each family member's unique cooperative response patterns.

CHAPTER 7

Co-constructing Change: Hosting Collaborative Conversations with Allies from Larger Systems

Out beyond ideas of wrongdoing and right doing there
is a field. I'll meet you there.

–RUMI

Once upon a time a North-Going Zax and a South-Going Zax met in the prairie of Prax. Much to their surprise, the two Zaxes came to a place where they ran into one another face to face. "Look here, now!" the North-Going Zax said. "I say! You are blocking my path. You are right in my way. I'm a North-Going Zax and I always go forth!" "Who is in whose way?" retorted the South-Going Zax. "I always go south, making south-going tracks so you're in My way!" This proved to be unacceptable to the North-Going Zax, who refused to budge and get out of the South-Going Zax's way. The North-Going Zax proclaimed that he would not move for "fifty-nine days!" The South-Going Zax countered with, "I can stand here in the prairie of Prax for fifty-nine years! I'll stay here, not budging! I can and I will if it makes you and me and the whole world stand still!" (Seuss, 1961b, pp. 27–31).

Dr. Seuss's *The Zax* is a nice metaphor for the kinds of interactions that can occur in collaborative meetings with those representatives from larger systems who are involved with our cases. Often, we and the helping professionals with whom we collaborate are not as forthright and assertive with one another about our opinions, assumptions, thoughts, and feelings as are the Zaxes. Instead, we tend to keep our private beliefs and opinions about cases to ourselves, which defeats the whole purpose of working together as a group to co-create possibilities for complex and challenging cases. Senge, Kleiner, Roberts, Ross, and Smith (1994, p. 242) have identified four ways our self-generating beliefs get us into trouble in collaborative meetings:

1. Our beliefs are the truth.
2. The truth is obvious.
3. Our beliefs are based on real data.
4. The data we select are the real data.

Therefore, to help combat these mental traps that can occur in collaborative meetings with helpers from larger systems and in our session with families, we can do the following: become more aware of our own thinking and reasoning, make our thinking and reasoning more visible to the helpers with whom we collaborate, and inquire into what the helpers' thinking and reasoning is in our collaborative conversations (Senge et al., 1994).

Not only is collaborating with helpers from larger systems a powerful and effective ecological approach for empowering families, but it is cost effective and supported by most managed care companies. Any treatment method that contributes to the rapid stabilization of the child's symptoms, helps prevent legal involvement, curtails school behavioral difficulties, and reduces the likelihood of psychiatric admissions will be given the Good Housekeeping Seal of Approval by managed care companies. Active and constructive collaboration with involved helping professionals can provide all of the above and more. When collaborative meetings are productive, the therapist working with the family and hosting the meetings is empowered as well. Doherty (1995) put it best when he said:

> Collaboration among professionals is the most clinician-friendly thing to do because it reduces professional isolation, enhances the knowledge and skills of all providers, and reduces the crushing sense of overresponsibility given the fact of one's own limited resources. (p. 276)

We become a "shared mind," which provides fertile soil for the generation of multiple high-quality solutions to resolve the child and family's difficulties rapidly.

In the remainder of this chapter, I discuss the role of the hosting therapist in family–multiple helper collaborative meetings, present key elements in successful collaborative relationships, and provide examples of collaborative questions that can be utilized in the context of these meetings. I follow with two case examples that illustrate the power of case collaboration.

ROLE OF THE HOSTING THERAPIST

Like all friendly and gracious hosts, we need to make visiting helpers feel warmly welcomed, and we must display good manners at all times. For some helping professionals, this kind of demeanor and way of relating comes as a pleasant surprise, especially if in the past therapists treated them as if they were the "enemy" or a "villain." It is my contention that we should adopt the view that each involved helping professional is a potential *ally* who possesses various strengths and resources that can help generate creative ideas for empowering the family. When we convey this therapeutic attitude to helping professionals, it greatly enhances cooperation and is the catalyst for building trust. The hosting therapist must demonstrate a deep respect for each helper's expertise, knowledge, skills, and varying perspectives on the case. According to McDaniel, Campbell, and Seaburn (1995), "Such behavior is like an engraved invitation that says, 'You may enter safely into my culture' " (p. 296).

After introductions have been made, each helping professional should be invited to share his or her story of involvement with the child and his or her family. Family members are free to comment on or provide feedback on any of the helpers' concerns or descriptions of them with which they disagree. For the family, this experience might be the first time in their long history of involvement with larger systems' representatives that they feel like they have a "voice" in their treatment. The hosting therapist's main job in the collaborative process with the helpers and the family is to be competent at keeping conversations going as long as possible, which can help generate new meanings about the problem story. He or she needs to operate from the Buddhist position of "Don't know mind" and utilize the therapeutic tool of *multipartiality* (Anderson & Goolishian, 1988b), that is, siding simultaneously with each family member's and helper's perspectives and not allowing his or her theoretical or personal views to dominate or take precedence.

If the hosting therapist in any way conveys a strong allegiance to a particular view or explanation, the flow of conversation can be shut down and quite possibly can alienate certain helpers attending the collaborative meeting. When we start parading our therapeutic views this way or behave with missionary zeal in the context of meetings, it can be useful to do the following: reflect on what was said in the collaborative process that made us anxious or put us on the defensive, ask open-ended conversational questions (Anderson & Goolishian, 1988a, 1988b, 1991a, 1991b), and be curious about what each helper is thinking or feeling about what was being discussed (McDaniel et al., 1995). The bottom line is, if we expect family members and involved helping professionals to be open to changing their problem-saturated views, we need to be equally ready and willing to change our views and behaviors. Hosting therapists can model this kind of flexibility by inviting helpers in their meetings to reflect on each others' views and by welcoming alternative viewpoints. We cannot escape from the reality that we are very much a part of the problem system. What we think and do can greatly influence the outcome of each family–multiple helper meeting.

As hosting therapists, we need to be sensitive to cultural differences (McDaniel et al., 1995) among the helping professionals participating in our meetings. For example, a psychiatrist speaks a much different language than a child protective worker. Both professionals have much different responsibilities and practice styles. We need to be respectful of the various helpers' cultural differences and the role of context in determining what they can hear and see. It is also helpful for the hosting therapist to converse in the helpers' differing languages, using their words and belief material about the case. When confused by certain words and their meaning, the hosting therapist should be a cultural anthropologist and ask the helper to explain what he or she means.

Finally, Peek and Heinrich (1995) stress that hosting therapists should "watch the team score, not just your own scores" (p. 338). When a case is in crisis or gets into trouble, so do all the helpers involved, even those doing a great job in their therapeutic area. It is crucial to be proactive and go the extra mile with more challenging or "stickier" cases in particular to prevent "case fractures and misunderstandings." This includes making phone calls and engaging in advocacy work between scheduled family–multiple helper collaborative meetings.

Out of respect for the family and the involved helpers' work schedules, we mutually decide the frequency of collaborative meetings and when they are scheduled. For absent helpers who were invited but could not attend, I have the family prepare a summary statement of what was discussed in a particular meeting, and we fax it or mail it to absent helpers so they are kept abreast of important new developments.

I also make myself available to meet with these helpers to discuss the case in their respective offices. The physical presence of all involved helping professionals in collaborative meetings is not necessary to create possibilities. (In point of fact, some of Einstein's most successful collaborations were by written correspondence with other scientists and scholars.) Sometimes, I put helpers who could not attend scheduled family–multiple helper meetings on the speaker box of the telephone so that they can call in from their car phone or offices and participate. In every way possible, I try to accommodate absent helpers, including scheduling future collaborative meetings at their offices so they can attend.

KEY ELEMENTS OF SUCCESSFUL COLLABORATIVE RELATIONSHIPS

Throughout history and across professional disciplines, one can find many examples of successful collaborative relationships. In fact, one study found that the majority of Nobel Prize winners had collaborated with an important colleague (e.g., Crick and Watson, the co-discoverers of the double helix theory of genetics). The famous Cubist painters George Braques and Pablo Picasso frequently advised each other as to whether or not a painting of the other's was completed (Schrage, 1990). In the arts, one highly successful collaborative relationship was that of lyricist Lorenz Hart and songwriter Richard Rodgers. Rodgers recalled:

> When the immovable object of his unwillingness to change came up against the irresistible force of my own drive for perfection . . . the noise could be heard all over the city. Our fights over words were furious, blasphemous, and frequent, but even in the hottest moments we both knew that we were arguing academically and not personally. (cited in Schrage, 1990, p. 41)

There are six key elements of successful collaborative relationships as applied to the context of family–multiple helper meetings.

There Is a Climate of Respect, Tolerance, and Trust

Every member of the family–multiple helper collaborative meeting must have a "voice" and be shown the utmost respect. The hosting therapist can model for collaborators *generative listening*, that is, not only listening to participants' words but to the very essence of his or her thinking, "the art of developing deeper silences in yourself" (Senge et al., 1994, p. 377). The hosting therapist also needs to model the importance of being nonjudgmental and suspending one's feelings (Isaacs, 1993). Each participant is treated as an equal and is given ample floor time to share his or her stories of concern about the family. Conversely, family members are free to be coauthors of their new evolving story without any participants serving as narrative editors and blocking them from having a "voice" in their own destiny and with treatment planning.

Communication Flow Is Flexible and Spontaneous

As mentioned earlier, the hosting therapist avoids providing too much structure for the family–multiple helper collaborative meetings. Besides kicking off the meeting with introductions and inviting helpers to share their stories of involvement with the family, the participants are given free reign to chime in at any point in the conversational process in the context of these meetings. During moments of silence after a participant speaks, it can be useful to try to generate some dialogue among participants or to make explicit our thoughts or reactions to what somebody said. When sharing our thoughts, they must be from a position of curiosity and with a suspension of disbelief, not coming across as wedded to one way of looking at things. At times, however, the hosting therapist may want to shift the group conversations away from focusing on what is not working and how to fix it and toward discovering and appreciating what is working with the child, his or her family, and the helpers involved, and how to leverage it. This can help create a "generative field" of mutual trust and appreciation, in which the group of helpers and the family will feel encouraged to discover and share their creative ideas and potential solutions (Brown & Isaacs, 1997; Cooperrider & Srivastva, 1987).

A Context Is Provided That Facilitates the Cross-Fertilization of Multiple Viewpoints

Ideally, the hosting therapist needs to co-create a context in which as many varying views of the problem story can be generated. By doing so, the involved helpers and family members begin to entertain new ways of looking at the problem-saturated situation and can coauthor new problem-free narratives. Physicist David Bohm refers to this process as a "stream of meaning" flowing among us, through us, and between us (Bohm, 1985). Once the involved helpers are less alarmed and concerned about the child and his or her family, because new understandings about the problem situation have been communicated and their view has changed, they will feel less compelled to have regular contact with the family and will eventually disengage from the problem system.

A Context Is Created That Plays with Multiple Viewpoints, Treating Uncertainty as an Opportunity for Further Exploration

When the hosting therapist brings together a roomful of helping providers with diverse health care and professional cultural backgrounds and a family entangled in the professional web, anything can happen and does. Sometimes our collaborations occur at the tops of our lungs. Sometimes there may be long silences and a strong sense of cautiousness in the air. In one meeting, several high-quality solutions may be generated by the group, or a family member may self-disclose the "not yet said" (Anderson & Goolishian, 1988b), which may be the missing piece of the family puzzle and may prove to be newsworthy to all participants. One never knows what shape or form these collaborative meetings will take. Einstein once said, "The most beautiful experience we can have is the mysterious. It is the fundamental emotion which stands at the cradle of true art and true science" (cited in Wujec, 1995, p. 27). The mysteriousness and uncertainty elements of these collaborative meetings are a constant reminder that knowledge is always on the way.

Consensus Is Not Necessary; It Is Irrelevant to the Act of Creation or Discovery

The fact that concensus is not necessary is elucidated in the collaborative relationship between Francis Crick and James Watson, co-developers of the double helix theory of genetics. According to Crick, "Politeness is the poison of all good collaboration in science" (cited in Schrage, 1990, p. 42). In describing the nature of his collaborative relationship with Watson, he had the following to say: "Our advantage was that we had evolved unstated but fruitful methods of collaboration.

... If either of us suggested a new idea, the other, while taking it seriously, would attempt to demolish it in a candid nonhostile manner" (cited in Schrage, 1990, p. 42). I am not suggesting or trying to convey that hosting therapists should behave this way with helpers in collaborative meetings, but it does demonstrate that we do not have to have group consensus to make important discoveries. We want to generate a kaleidoscopic view of the problem story which is more likely to lead to opening up the door to creating new possibilities. Also, by avoiding the push for group consensus, we are modeling for family members that there are many ways to look at their problem situation, none more "correct" than others. This can help loosen up fixed beliefs that family members have had about the identified child client and the helpers who have been involved in their lives.

There Are No Restrictive Boundaries Regarding Who Does What

One of the most beautiful and common occurrences in the context of family–multiple helper collaborative meetings are the spontaneous offers by participating providers to advocate for and assist family members in the various social contexts in which they had been experiencing difficulties. For example, one school social worker who was participating in a collaborative meeting I was hosting spontaneously offered to advocate for and help the identified child client resolve a long-standing conflict with a particular teacher who was known to be "difficult." I had not suggested in any way that the school social worker intervene on the child's behalf; she came up with this idea spontaneously. As a result of her efforts, the child began to view her as a "caring" ally in the school who was available to him, and she became instrumental in helping him resolve the conflict problem with the so-called difficult teacher. This example demonstrates the hosting therapist need not assign tasks or responsibilities to participants in the collaborative meetings. Once participating helpers begin to feel like their knowledge and expertise is respected, they will begin to take more positive risks, such as offering to go the extra mile for families.

COLLABORATIVE INTERVIEWING

The hosting therapist has to be a good diplomat, translator, and master conversationalist. As a key meaning maker in the collaborative process, he or she models the importance of being curious about the second and third possible explanation for the problem story and asks questions from a position of "not knowing" rather than "pre-knowing" (Anderson & Goolishian, 1988b). Lao-tzu, author of the *Tao Te Ching*, offered the following words of wisdom about the dangers of adopting a pre-knowing stance: "The more you know, the less you understand" (cited in Mitchell, 1988, p. 47). Therefore, the hosting therapist needs to ask open-ended conversational questions (Andersen, 1991, 1995; Anderson & Goolishian, 1988a, 1988b), which help enlarge meaning about the continually evolving problem story. At the same time, the hosting therapist should not hesitate to make his or her thinking and reasoning known to all participants in the meeting, being careful not to offend anyone and "honoring the passion" that underlies their varying view-points (Senge et al., 1994).

I now present some examples of the types of collaborative questions I may ask family members and helpers in the context of our meetings together, followed by a brief discussion on the importance of the therapist's use of self-reflexive questions.

Collaborative Questions

Collaborative questions are open-ended and the hosting therapist's primary tool in the meaning-making process. Such questions contribute to the restorying process, which ultimately leads to the authoring of new and more preferred family narratives: Examples of collaborative questions include the following:

> "Let's say that this group of providers, including myself, proved to be most helpful to you [the family], what sort of things would we have done that benefited you the most?"
>
> "What led you to that way of seeing things?"
>
> "What do you mean by that view?"
>
> "You may be right, but I'd like to understand more. What leads you to believe . . . ?"
>
> "If you [the family] were conducting this meeting, what do you think all of us providers really need to know about this problem situation and your family?"
>
> "What are your thoughts about why this problem exists?"
>
> "How did you first get involved with this family?"

"What is your present role in this family's life?"

"What ideas do you have about this problem situation?"

"What are you most concerned about?"

"Once that problem is resolved, will you continue to be involved with this family?"

"When you said that, what did you mean?"

"Is there something that needs to be talked about that we have not touched on as yet?"

"What has kept that issue from not being talked about?"

Self-Reflexive Questions

Self-reflexive questions (Bohm, 1996; Schon, 1983; Senge et al., 1994) can aid hosting therapists in paying closer attention to how their own emotional reactions, beliefs, and opinions block them from being totally open to all possible viewpoints that are generated in the context of family–multiple helper meetings. All hosting therapists and participating helpers bring to collaborative meetings assumptions about the child cases with which they are mutually involved. Our assumptions can block us from truly hearing what others are saying and from entertaining new ways at looking at a case. According to Bohm (1996) we need to "suspend our assumptions, so that we neither act on them nor suppress them. Suspension is helpful in that it creates a mirror so that you can see the results of your thought" (p. 25). We can ask ourselves these questions as a form of private dialogue in the process of meetings or when reflecting to ourselves immediately after meetings. Examples of self-reflexive questions include the following:

"What has really led me to think and feel this way?"

"How might my comments have contributed to the difficulties in our meeting?"

"What unhelpful assumptions am I making about [particular providers]?"

"What were my intentions in this meeting?"

"What prevented me from behaving differently?"

"By having this meeting, did I achieve the results I was intending?"

"What difference did this meeting make for the family?"

"As a result of this meeting, did the family appear to leave feeling empowered, or did it not seem to make much of a difference to them?"

"If I had an opportunity to replay this whole meeting over again, what would I have done differently as the host facilitator?"

CASE EXAMPLES

A Case of the LD Blues

Victoria Smith brought her 11-year-old son, Sebastian, in for therapy for his "aggressive behavior" toward peers, "poor grades," and "low self-esteem" because of his "learning disability" problem. The Catholic school that Sebastian attended had threatened to kick him out because of his "aggressive tendencies," "mischievous ways," and "failing grades." The Smiths had been to "five therapists" prior to seeing me. Victoria was convinced that Sebastian's behavioral difficulties were "at the root" of his "feeling of inadequacy" caused by his alleged "visual perceptual processing deficit," which had been "identified through testing by the district psychologist" when Sebastian was in third grade. Victoria's key question for years had been: "Has the visual perceptual processing deficit caused Sebastian's low self-esteem?" When exploring past treatment experiences with Victoria, she made it quite clear to me that none of the former therapists could "provide answers" to her question, nor could they develop a "relationship with Sebastian." In some ways the latter problem became a negative self-fulfilling prophecy that had been perpetrated with every new therapist. I, too, experienced great difficulty in getting in the door with Sebastian. He refused to say a word to me, even when I met with him alone. The use of humor and the miracle question (de Shazer, 1988) proved to be futile with Sebastian. By the end of the session, the best I could do was ask Victoria to experiment by "not mentioning a word about school to Sebastian for a whole week." She had agreed that "hounding him daily about doing his homework" tended to lead to "arguments" and made matters worse. After conducting a macrosystemic assessment with the family, Victoria was eager for me to talk with Sebastian's teachers, the school principal, and their pediatrician, who was also concerned about Sebastian's situation. Victoria and Sebastian signed the consent forms so that I could collaborate with the school personnel and the pediatrician.

As my office was not too far away from the school, the art, gym, and homeroom teachers agreed to come there for our first collabora- tive meeting with Victoria and Sebastian. Because of scheduling prob- lems, neither the school principal nor the pediatrician could attend this first meeting in person but agreed to be put on the speaker box at staggered times. After brief introductions, I invited each of the helpers to share their stories of involvement and concerns about Sebastian. In the school context, only the homeroom teacher had some positive things to say. Despite Sebastian's "testy" behavior at times, the homeroom teacher shared that she thought Sebastian possessed "excel- lent assertiveness skills" and was a "natural-born leader." I noticed that a slight smile appeared on Sebastian's face after his homeroom teacher acknowledged his strengths.

In responding to Sebastian's nonverbal response, I asked him whether he thought his homeroom teacher wanted to "join his fan club." For the first time, I got Sebastian to laugh and respond. He pointed out that he liked his homeroom teacher the most. Suddenly, the art teacher voiced a strong desire to "join Sebastian's fan club" as well. Sebastian appeared very surprised by his art teacher's response. He asked her, "Why would you want to join? I'm getting an F in your class." The art teacher responded by complimenting Sebastian on his "artistic abilities when he applies himself." She also pointed out some ways that Sebastian could "pick up" his grade. Despite the positive interactions between Sebastian and two of his teachers, this was not newsworthy to the gym teacher or the principal. Although the gym teacher began by complimenting Sebastian on his "athletic abilities," he switched gears to tell how Sebastian was a "big troublemaker" and often "does not follow the rules." The principal chimed in that there is "no other child" he "sees more" in his office than Sebastian. Sebastian cried out, "You never have anything good to say about me!" Victoria defended her son and put the principal on the spot by asking him to give her son "a chance" and "stop beating his self-es- teem down all of the time." The principal was silent for a few minutes and made it clear that he didn't like "playing the heavy" and "would love" to see a reduction in Sebastian's visits to his office. Sebastian pointed out that he didn't like to have to visit the principal either. Finally, the pediatrician had nothing but praise for Sebastian's talents and good qualities.

We scheduled a follow-up meeting 4 weeks later. The mother hugged and kissed Sebastian at the end of the meeting and told him how proud she was of him. Both the art and homeroom teachers patted Sebastian on the back and said they would help him in any way they could. The Smiths and I decided to not to meet until our next collaborative meeting.

Four weeks later, we met as a group at the school. The pediatrician could not attend because of his hectic schedule. Across the board, the multiple helpers had only glorious reports about Sebastian's behavior. The district psychologist had retested Sebastian and reported in our meeting that he could not find any signs of learning deficits or problem areas for concern. All the teachers reported that Sebastian was "well behaved," "cooperative," and "showed good self-control" when provoked by peers. Both the gym teacher and the principal were astonished by Sebastian's complete behavioral turnaround. Victoria pointed out that his behavior had improved at home and he seemed "much happier these days." We all agreed that we could hold off scheduling another meeting because Sebastian had made tremendous progress behaviorally and academically. I ended up seeing the family two more times, and therapy was successfully concluded.

As a result of the family–multiple helper meetings, new narratives were generated about Sebastian's alleged learning disability/deficit (LD) handicap and being perceived as the big troublemaker at school. An alternative, preferred story was coauthored in our first collaborative meeting that described Sebastian as being a natural-born leader, being artistic, possessing excellent assertiveness skills, and having good athletic abilities. Sebastian was empowered by our meetings and did a nice job of asserting himself, which challenged his mother's long-standing belief that her son was "paralyzed emotionally" by his "low self-esteem." It was also a newsworthy experience for me to witness the spontaneous and assertive sides to Sebastian.

A Little Daredevil

Cedric, a 10-year-old African American boy, was court-referred for treatment because of his long history of "shoplifting" from "toy stores" and such school behavioral problems as "mouthing-off" to teachers and other school personnel and "stealing from students." Cedric had been adopted by the Hineses when he was 3 years old. The adoptive parents knew very little about Cedric's biological parents. Because they were unable to bear their own children, they were thrilled to get Cedric. However, they described Cedric as being "difficult to raise since day one" and as always being "a little daredevil." Cedric was constantly testing their limits and throwing "temper tantrums," and he began stealing from them at the age of 8. "Yelling at him" and "taking his toys away" proved to be futile in curtailing those behaviors, which continued to the present day. In school, he was constantly in the principal's office, which eventually led to his being placed in a behavior-disordered (BD) program in the school district. According to the parents, Cedric associated with "older" peers in the neighborhood who were "up to no good." One time, the mother came home after work and found Cedric and these "older boys" on the roof of their house. Finally, Cedric had been caught a few times by store security guards trying to steal "Game Boy" computer toys. The last time Cedric got caught, the store owner pressed charges.

Cedric was tough and very precocious. He acted more like a 16-year-old. He appeared to be very street smart and shared with me when I met with him alone that he mainly hung out with older kids in their midteens. I asked Cedric how I could be helpful to him. Cedric's main complaints were that his parents always went through his "bedroom drawers looking for things" and his probation officer made "surprise visits" to his house and school. I played Columbo with Cedric and asked, "What could your parents possibly be looking for in your bedroom?" He responded with, "Oh ... Game Boys." I shared with Cedric how confused I was about what he did with all the Game Boys he had taken. I asked him if he stole them for friends or sold them for money. Cedric was quite open with me and reported that he did both. We related well with one another talking about how much each of us liked Michael Jordan and the Chicago Bulls basketball team.

After reconvening with the family, I explored their thoughts on whom I needed to collaborate with. The parents suggested the probation officer, the school social worker, the principal, and their church pastor, who was very concerned about Cedric's behavioral problems. Family members signed the appropriate consent forms. The initial treatment goals were for the parents to experiment with "not going through Cedric's bedroom drawers for a week." Cedric agreed to reconnect with a friend his own age and "stay away" from the "older friends" with whom he tended to get into trouble. I also shared with Cedric that I would help get his "probation officer off his back." Cedric was happy that I was willing to help him out with the probation officer. Because I had a good working relationship with the probation officer, I could easily negotiate with him to help my clients.

Present at our first collaborative meeting were Cedric, his parents, the school social worker, the probation officer, and the pastor. The principal made it quite clear to me on the telephone that he had already "wiped his hands clean of Cedric" and had no time to attend after-school meetings. After everyone shared their stories of involvement with this case, the pastor began with a minisermon about how worried he was about Cedric's "ending up in a street gang" if he didn't change. The parents chimed in that they thought it might already be "too late by the looks of some of the older boys Cedric runs with." Cedric took a risk with the group and disclosed that he used to run with "Anthony and Leon" who were both members of the "Disciples" street gang. He had cut off contact with them because they used "drugs" and "beat up" kids in the neighborhood. Out of curiosity I asked Cedric if Anthony and Leon had anything to do with his stealing Game Boys. Again, Cedric took a risk with me and the group and disclosed that they had threatened to "kick" his "ass" if he didn't steal for them. This information proved to be quite newsworthy to all the participants in our meeting. They had no idea that Cedric was being "bullied to steal for the gang members." Out of concern, the probation officer offered to intervene on Cedric's behalf with the two gang members. He also shared his plan to "let the judge know the truth" about Cedric's "shoplifting" situation at the next court date. Cedric thanked the probation officer and shared with the whole group how "scared" he had been about "getting caught stealing" and the gang's coming after him if he would "quit doing this" for them. The school social worker and the parents offered to help out with support and protection. For added protection, the pastor offered to hook Cedric up with an African American community leader who was respected by the street gangs. He also pointed out to the group that Jesse, the community leader, "coached a basketball team" for kids around Cedric's age. Cedric got excited about this and left our meeting more hopeful and in good spirits. The next scheduled collaborative meeting was for 6 weeks later.

During the interval break, I saw Cedric and his family twice. The parents reported that Cedric was being a "good boy" and "following" their "rules" and had "stopped stealing." Another important change was that the parents "did not receive one call from the school" about Cedric's problem behavior. Cedric also met Jesse and began attending his basketball practices to help "keep him off the streets."

Six weeks later, I met with all of the helpers, the Hines family, and Jesse. Across the board, all the helpers and Jesse had glowing reports to give about Cedric's progress. The parents also shared in front of the whole group how pleased they were with Cedric's progress. Mrs. Hines brought a large cake that she had baked for the group as a token of her appreciation for all of their "kindness" and "help" with Cedric. Even the school principal, who was originally so skeptical and pessimistic about Cedric's ability to change, became a true believer that the "new responsible Cedric" was here to stay. We mutually agreed to meet one more time as a group in 3 months.

I ended up seeing Cedric and his family four more times over a 6-month period. Cedric's behavior continued to improve both at home and at school. His mother no longer referred to him as a little daredevil; instead, she used the words "responsible young man" to describe him. Cedric had become one of Jesse's "star" basketball players. Cedric also got let off court supervision 3 months earlier than the judge originally ordered because of his tremendous progress.

As readers can clearly see, by actively collaborating with the involved helpers in the child's social ecology, rapid and quite dramatic changes can occur in one or more group meetings. Doing and thinking ecologically can make treatment much more efficient and effective. Margaret Mead summed it up best when she said: "Never doubt that a small group of committed citizens can change the world, indeed, it is the only thing that ever does" (cited in Vandenberg, 1993, p. 91).

CHAPTER 8

"Impossible" Cases: From Therapeutic Breakthroughs to Treatment Failures

I have not failed. I have merely found 10,000 ways that won't work.

–Thomas Edison

From time to time, we all are assigned or referred cases that become our worst nightmares. These "impossible" family cases are analogous to trying to find our way out of a maze in a dark room. Not all "impossible" cases start off being impossible. Sometimes things are going very well early in treatment and then, all of a sudden, the case takes a turn for the worse. Even after our best efforts to consolidate gains, the case falls apart. It is easy to tell when we are faced with an "impossible" case. Some common symptoms experienced by therapists are feeling frustrated or angry with particular family members, fantasizing about the family's failing to show up for appointments, dreading having to see the family, canceling appointments with them at the last minute, frenetically searching for the "utopian" solutions or interventions for the family, and being stuck doing "more of the same" (Watzlawick et al., 1974) with the family. With some impossible cases, no matter what we do or don't do, treatment is a failure.

In this chapter, I present several different therapeutic pathways that therapists can pursue with stuck or challenging cases that are "impossible," "resistant," "difficult," and "our worst nightmare." I also discuss the importance of failing with family cases once in awhile and the valuable wisdom we can gain from these therapeutic experiences.

USE OF THE CHILD'S "PAL"
AS AN EXPERT CONSULTANT

Little research has been conducted on the importance of children's relationships in social skills development and the long-lasting effects of these early relationships on the ability to build and sustain relationships later in life. One longitudinal study on children's relationships found the following: They provide opportunities for learning social skills, help the child feel a sense of belonging to a group, and contribute to self-acceptance, identity, and the ability to trust others (Cowen, Pederson, Babigian, Izzo, & Trost, 1973).

No other theorist and psychotherapist has examined more the significance of children's relationships, particularly the child's relationship with his or her "chum," than Harry Stack Sullivan (Rubin, 1980; Cottrell & Foote, 1995). Sullivan referred to this chum as being a "fortunate someone" of the child's same sex with whom an unprecedented degree of intimacy could occur. He believed the child and his or her chum could communicate on equal terms, exchange a vast amount of ideas and information with one another, compare notes, and develop sympathy for each other when faced with life's stressors (Cottrell & Foote, 1995).

In three earlier publications (Selekman, 1991, 1993, 1995b), I wrote about several different ways therapists could utilize adolescent clients' friends in family therapy. The friends can be employed as expert consultants in sessions, as a natural support system in larger social contexts in which the identified client is experiencing difficulties, and as valuable resources in family–multiple helper collaborative meetings. The challenging case of a very bright 10-year-old boy who was experiencing a great deal of peer rejection and harassment demonstrates how the use of a child's pal as an expert consultant in family therapy sessions not only can help unstick the treatment system but can serve as a catalyst for child and family changes.

> Chuck was brought in for therapy by his parents, who were quite concerned about his "poor peer relations," "low self-esteem," "depression," and "isolating a lot in his bedroom." Also, Chuck's "grades were slipping." Despite Chuck's great difficulty in being accepted by peers, he had one close pal, Bill, with whom he grew up. Bill was "popular" both at school and in the neighborhood. He was a "talented athlete," an "excellent student," and a "very sensitive and caring boy." According to the parents, Bill frequently provided "moral support" for Chuck, particularly when the kids at

school or in the neighborhood "teased him" and physically "pushed him around." Chuck's peers often called him a "dork" because he was very uncoordinated and performed poorly in sports activities. Bill accompanied the family to this first family interview but did not participate.

When meeting alone with the parents, I learned that they had experienced failure in family therapy three times before. The mother cited Chuck's refusal to talk in sessions with the therapists as the main reason for past failures in family therapy. The parents were hard-pressed to give me any advice about how I could get in the door with Chuck. Their key question about the problem situation was, "Why is Chuck behaving this way?" I normalized Chuck's behaviors as resulting from peer rejection and harassment. This explanation about the problem appeared to be helpful for the parents, especially how peer rejection at this age and older can wreak havoc on a child's self-esteem.

My individual session time with Chuck was not as productive. No matter what I said or did, Chuck would either utter one-word responses or not respond at all. Humor and offers to play cards or board games went absolutely nowhere. When I asked the miracle question (de Shazer, 1988) earlier in the session, Chuck was similarly silent. While on an intersession break, I decided to present the idea to Chuck and his parents of including Bill in our next family session in a participatory role. Because Bill had such a close relationship with Chuck, I thought he could be a helpful consultant for the family and me in future sessions. At this point, I was ready and willing to try anything, as I had been unable to negotiate a well-formed goal with the family or to come up with any therapeutic tasks to offer them. Both the parents and Chuck agreed to try including Bill in the next session. Chuck's parents were friendly with Bill's parents and planned to talk to Bill's parents about our idea.

In our second family session, I decided to capitalize as much as possible on Bill's expertise. I explored with Bill whether he had any helpful advice for Chuck's parents on what they could do to help Chuck out. Bill recommended that the parents "stop trying to push Chuck to go out" all the time. He pointed out that when he pushes Chuck to do things, Chuck "gets mad" and "won't do" what Bill wants him to do. The parents were surprised to hear that Bill was experiencing the same difficulty with Chuck. I asked Bill, if he were Chuck's dad, what he would do instead to get Chuck out of his bedroom more. Bill recommended that the father should offer to play a computer game with Chuck. Apparently, Bill and Chuck often played computer games together. At this point in the session, I asked Chuck what he thought of Bill's suggestions so far. Chuck said he would feel "happier" if his parents did what Bill suggested. I then asked Bill for any advice for me as a therapist in how to best help Chuck out. Bill encouraged me not to ask a "lot of questions" and to avoid pushing Chuck as the parents had been doing. Chuck chimed in for the first time and responded, "Yeah, don't be like my parents . . . I would have played chess with you if you would have given me some time!" By the end of our session, we were all in agreement that Bill had been very helpful to all of us and was free to come back for future sessions. I asked Bill what his consultation fee was before we closed out the meeting. Bill and the parents laughed and Bill promised not to charge me for his time.

I ended up seeing the family four more times after our second session. In the third and fourth sessions, I employed Bill's services when teaching Chuck assertiveness skills to help him better deal with difficult peers. Bill role-played the difficult peer role with Chuck so Chuck could practice assertiveness skills. They also switched roles, which proved enlightening to Chuck in terms of learning more about himself in social situations. Finally, to further empower Chuck when he was harassed and rejected by peers, I provided cognitive skills training (Seligman, 1995). To help Chuck combat negative thoughts and his tendency to catastrophize, I taught him how to search for evidence to support his irrational thoughts, as well as to visualize in his mind's eye a stop light turning red to help disrupt the unhelpful thought patterns. The combination of Bill's expert advice and support and the cognitive skills training helped Chuck and his family resolve their difficulties quickly. Chuck's grades improved and he learned effective tools for being less reactive to peer harassment and rejection. Chuck became friends with another boy his age who lived on his block. The parents also implemented Bill's most helpful suggestion of "backing off" and "not pushing Chuck" to go out more. By our last session, they reported that Chuck appeared to have "higher self-esteem" and was no longer "depressed."

ADVENTURES IN PARENTING: TEACHING PARENTS NEW DANCE STEPS

With some of the more challenging family cases, the parents may be stuck in a *same* or *worse* cooperative response pattern of relating to the therapist. Their response pattern thus becomes rigidified and does not respond well to the use of externalization of the problem (White, 1995; White & Epston, 1990), family play and art therapy tasks, or the Solution-Focused therapeutic tasks (de Shazer, 1985, 1988, 1991) described in Chapter 4. I have witnessed a number of cases in which the parents were stuck in superresponsible positions or power struggles with their children, and even the Do Something Different task (de Shazer, 1985) failed to produce any significant changes in altering their children's problematic behaviors. Perhaps the parents' choices of doing things differently around the child were too similar to their past attempts, or they failed to go beyond the threshold level that kept the problem-maintaining pattern intact.

Parents, like therapists, often take their jobs way too seriously and forget about how to lighten up or about the joys of having fun with their children. Often, parents will describe their children's problems as enormous mountains before them, blocking them from seeing the times when their children are engaging in positive, prosocial behaviors. No question, being a parent is a tough job, and even the best of parents fall into the rut of engaging in habitual "more of the same" (Watzlawick et al., 1974) dances with their children, which inadvertently end up reinforcing the very behaviors they want to eliminate. For example, I remember when I would try to rush my daughter Hanna to get dressed in the morning so I could get her ready to go to day care and I could go to my job. The more I pressured her to get dressed, the more she would say "no!" and continue to rebel. In this situation, I missed the fact that we cannot box young children into adult schedules. Finally, one day, by having a conversation with Hanna's Winnie the Pooh figurine about what clothes she should wear for the day, I found a solution that worked. Hanna came running into her bedroom and stood right next to me, listening intently to what Winnie the Pooh and I were talking about. I had Winnie the Pooh point out to Hanna her potential clothing options. It was Winnie the Pooh's decision to let Hanna choose what clothing combination she would wear for the day. Through the use of parental improvisation and imagination, I found a high-quality solution that worked for me in "the getting Hanna dressed" department. In fact, I met with equal success in using this strategy to distract Hanna from temper tantrums and cranky behavior.

Parenting experts would agree that there is no substitute for giving children daily "special attention time" (Forehand & Long, 1996; Rosemond, 1994; Taffel, 1991). Parents need to protect this special time from being disrupted by outside influences or other responsibilities. By giving children this daily special time, they feel valued, important, and nurtured. The child needs to be put in the driver's seat to determine what he or she would like to talk about or do during this special time. Some working parents get so caught up in the hustle and bustle of their work lives that their interactions with their children are of the negative variety, that is, yelling or quite visibly looking stressed out most of the time during the week. I recommend that such parents set aside a designated amount of time daily or whenever necessary to spend with the child or children.

In this section, I present three parental strategies that can be utilized with parents who are stuck doing more of the same (Watzlawick et al., 1974) and provide case examples.

Novel and Surprising Tactics

I point out to parents who are habitually stuck in power struggles with their child that the more they end up in center ring sparring with the child the more the child will win. Often these parents do not recognize that the more out of control they get, the more their child will escalate and get equally out of control. This becomes a "game without an end" (Watzlawick et al., 1974). Similar to the rationale I give to parents when I prescribe the Do Something Different task (de Shazer, 1985), I let the parents know that they are far too predictable in their child's mind, and the best way they can win back control over their child in a positive and fun way is to present themselves to him or her in novel and surprising ways. Most parents tend to smile and warm up to experimenting with this new way of interacting with their child, particularly when they are feeling so frustrated and at their wits' end with the problem situation. Before sending the parents off to try this new parenting experiment, I brainstorm with them what ideas they have regarding novel and surprising things they could try with the child. I once worked with some parents who surprised their strong-willed and difficult 9-year-old son by walking around the house dressed in Halloween costumes for a few days. The son was so perplexed by the parents' bizarre behavior that he began to cooperate more with the directives and expectations. As part of this discussion, I share some creative things other parents have done that proved to be quite successful, such as rolling around on the living room floor hugging and kissing each other while the child was throwing a big temper tantrum or starting to dance in a strange manner when the child was being disrespectful to them. In both of these case scenarios, the parents were quickly able to curtail their children's temper tantrum and oppositional behavior problems by using these novel and surprising tactics. The following case example of an 8-year-old girl illustrates the effectiveness of parents employing novel and surprising behaviors to change their child's behaviors.

> Amber was brought in for therapy because of her "violent tendencies," oppositional behavior, and "aggressive" behavior toward her mother, Linda, and 3-year-old sister, Belle. Amber's parents had been divorced for 4 years. Linda had divorced Amber's biological father because he was "violent" and "screamed a lot." He was also described as an "alcoholic." Linda pointed out that her ex-husband was very inconsistent with visitations. Amber rarely talked about her father. Belle was a product of Linda's new "serious relationship" with Tom, her fiancé. Tom and Amber got along well. Linda described Amber as being a "holy terror." When she got angry, Amber had a tendency to "break her toys," "scream," and "push and punch" Linda. At times, she would "torment" Belle. For the first two sessions, Linda came alone with Amber. One big exception reported by Linda was Amber's academic prowess, for she was an A student. Neither Linda nor Amber's teacher could explain why Amber's behavior was "perfect" in school. It was only at home that Amber was experiencing serious behavioral problems. It was clear that Linda was at her wits' end in trying to gain Amber's compliance and reduce her aggressive behaviors.
>
> In our first two sessions, I failed to engage Amber. She kept her distance from me, refused to play board games, and displayed little interest in doing a family art task with her mother. According to Linda, it took time for Amber to "warm up to strangers." Because Linda spent most of the session complaining about Amber, I decided to give her an observation task to assist us in identifying exceptions that we could use as building blocks for solution construction. I also suggested that we include Tom in our next session because the exceptions Linda observed in Amber's behavior were not newsworthy to her and Amber's behavior was not changing.
>
> I spent the majority of the third session alone with Linda and Tom. I proposed to them that we experiment with novel, surprising parental behaviors over the next week. Neither Linda nor Tom could come up with any ideas that they thought would make a difference in altering Amber's difficult behaviors. I recommended that they experiment with "kissing and hugging and rolling around on the floor every time Amber pushed their buttons." I also encouraged the couple to try to come up with their own unique

off-the-wall behaviors to surprise Amber. The couple smiled and appeared eager to test out the experiment.

One week later, the couple came back reporting that Amber's behavior had greatly improved. Amber asked me what I had done to her parents. She described them as acting "strange." I shared with Amber that "sometimes parents act strange when they try too hard to be the best parents they can be." Amber hugged her mother and told her that she did not have to "try so hard" because she loved her. When I met alone with the parents, they were smiling and laughing about how much fun they were having with the experiment. I recommended that they continue to do more of what was working. Because of their progress, I gave the family a vacation from therapy as a vote of confidence.

I ended up seeing the family four more times to consolidate gains, teach other parenting skills, and help Amber learn more effective ways to express her anger and frustration with her mother. Once the parents changed their dance steps around Amber in a novel and surprising way, we were better able to do some productive work together as a family. Another important change was Amber's self-disclosure about her angry feelings about her biological father's rejection. Both Linda and Tom provided Amber with a lot of support around this painful issue. Recognizing that the biological father was very much a part of the problem system, I tried several times to engage him for family sessions; however, he failed either to show up for appointments or to return my telephone calls. Despite his refusal to work with us, we were successfully able to resolve Amber's problems with aggressive and oppositional behavior. The power in using novel and surprising tactics with stuck parents is that it helps them see how their routine and automatic reasoning and "more of the same" attempted solutions are getting them into trouble. Parents often also report improvements in their self-reflection and problem-solving skills as a result of experimenting with novel and surprising tactics.

Positive Consequences

One highly effective way for parents to increase the likelihood of prosocial and cooperative behaviors with their children is to utilize *positive consequences* with the children when they misbehave. Some examples of positive consequences are as follows: being given a desig-nated amount of time to construct and write a card for a relative, finding two lawns in the neighborhood to mow (for older children), doing one good deed for a neighbor, and devoting a whole weekend day to one parent to assist him or her with household projects. Parents can be as creative as they want to be in selecting the positive consequence. It is most important, however, that the positive consequence selected contributes to building the child's sense of self-worth, teaches the importance of being responsible, and benefits others.

Like novel and surprising parental tactics, having parents give their children positive consequences teaches them new dance steps which can promote more behavioral compliance and improve the quality of their parent–child relationships. This parental strategy is particularly useful for parents who are stuck frequently punishing their children, giving extreme and lengthy punishments for misbehavior, or viewing the child's misbehavior as a personal assault on them—"He's doing this deliberately to make me angry!" According to leading parenting experts, excessive use of punishment can lead to a child's dislike, resentment, and aggression toward his or her parents (Forehand & Long, 1996; Greenspan, 1995; Taffel, 1991). In their research, Forehand and Long (1996) found that "parents who use excessive punishment frequently find themselves on the receiving end of their child's indignation" (p. 19). Taffel (1991) contends that punishment often does not "fit the crime." He argues that taking away a child's highly prized toy or computer for 1 month as punishment for misbehaving is "downright illogical." Along these same lines, Seligman (1995) stresses that parents should "indict only the specific action, not the child" (p. 289). It is not the child who is bad; it is the action that is bad. The following case example illustrates how teaching parents the value of positive consequences helped them move away from screaming, engaging in needless power struggles, and resorting to brute force with their strong-willed, highly oppositional 10-year-old boy.

> Jimmy was brought for therapy because of his "total disrespect" of his parents' "rules," not responding to their "consequences," constantly "talking back" to his mother, and having behavioral problems in school. I discovered early in the first session that I was the sixth therapist the parents had taken Jimmy to see. The parents made it quite clear to me that if I failed to help Jimmy, they would try to get him "residentially placed." To try to create possibilities in the session, I asked the miracle question (de Shazer, 1988); however, the parents quickly told me that they didn't "believe in miracles." The more I tried to cooperate with the parents' pessimism, the more pessimistic they became with their responses.

Jimmy sat apart from us with his head down and refused to respond to my questions. When I asked the parents open-ended conversational questions (Andersen, 1995; Anderson & Goolishian, 1988a, 1989) to give them plenty of room to tell their long, problem-saturated story, they continued to blame Jimmy for "all the stress" in their "lives."

I dismissed Jimmy from the room and met alone with the parents. I asked them to give me a videotape-like description of a recent problem scenario with Jimmy. Apparently, the mother had asked Jimmy to put his dirty dishes in the dishwasher. Jimmy "cussed" his mother out and she "slapped him in the face." She then told him to "go to his room," but he refused to budge from the chair he was sitting in, in front of the TV. The father then "lifted Jimmy out of his seat" and literally "carried him" to his bedroom "kicking and screaming." After an hour of carrying on, Jimmy eventually quieted down and went to sleep. According to the parents, this was an atypical scenario; tempers had never flared this badly before.

It was clear that the parents were feeling frustrated and stuck, unable to come up with consequences that would work with Jimmy. They were finding that "taking his stereo away" for long periods of time, "yelling," and "not letting him out of the house after school" only added fuel to Jimmy's oppositional and recalcitrant behavior. The mother felt "guilty" for striking Jimmy and vowed that she would "not let this happen again." As the parents appeared ready to move from being complainants into customers, I proposed we experiment with implementing the positive consequences strategy. Although the parents had their doubts that this parenting strategy could work, they were willing to test it out. I predicted that they would struggle with avoiding the temptations to yell, to think that Jimmy was going out of his way to frustrate them, and to cave in to wanting to take things away from him. My individual session time with Jimmy proved to be futile, as he refused to talk with me or engage in any activity with me.

The parents came in alone the following week with a good progress report. They had allowed Jimmy to go to a hockey game with a friend's family because he had had a much better week. They found that by being calmer and firmer and giving Jimmy positive consequences, he responded better to their limits. One night Jimmy had "talked back" to his mother, so she had him "wash two loads of clothes" as a consequence for "mouthing off" to her.

When Jimmy failed to straighten up his bedroom as requested by his father, his father had him pick up all the scraps of paper and other garbage in their flower beds and around their house. Jimmy also straightened up his bedroom the next day.

I ended up seeing the family six more times. Simply changing the parents' dance steps and outmoded beliefs about Jimmy led to Jimmy's becoming more compliant and prosocial. We also implemented the positive consequences strategy at school with Jimmy's main teacher. Rather than sending him down to the principal's office all the time, the teacher would arrange tasks for Jimmy to do around the school. The teacher found that the positive consequences strategy helped improve Jimmy's behavior in the class room.

Taking a Trip to Parentland

The use of imagination and guided fantasy with parents can be quite effective at moving them out of the "black box" into new parental realities with their children. One imagination task I frequently utilize with parents is Taking a Trip to Parentland. The in-session task begins with the following questions:

> "Suppose you were to wake up tomorrow and find yourselves in Parentland, where parents are totally fulfilled by their important roles, are regarded by society as its most important citizens, and have well-behaved children, what would you observe these parents doing for themselves and their children that makes them feel so fulfilled as parents?"

> "What effect would those things appear to have on how these parents feel about themselves and interact with their children?"

> "What are those parents doing for themselves as a couple individually that seems to enhance their parenting abilities the most?"

> "What specifically are those parents doing with their children that appears to foster good behavior?"

> "If you were to bring back two things you learned from the parents in Parentland that you would want to implement with your own children, what would they be?"

> "What else would you do differently with your children?"

Helping stuck and frustrated parents gain some distance from their problem situations and approach their challenging jobs from different angles can empower them to be more flexible and effective in managing their children. In the following case example, all my clinical work was with the parents.

> Roberta and Carlo, an Italian couple, came to our clinic seeking advice about how to resolve their 9-year-old daughter, Mia's, "chronic lying" problem. Mia had been lying to her parents since age 6. The parents had "no clue" about why Mia continued to lie to them "about everything." "Everything" included the following: "sneaking food" out of the kitchen, "secretly" associating with a "troublemaking" peer in the neighborhood, and "lying about grades" she received on school papers and tests. The parents attempted solutions had been "yelling," lecturing, taking Mia's stereo and TV out of her bedroom, and "not allowing her to go out" and play after school. Both parents were feeling so frustrated with Mia that they began to think that she was "deliberately lying" to make them "mad." Because the parents presented themselves as complainants, I decided to give them an observation task of keeping track of the times when Mia was not lying to them and what they were doing that helped promote this prosocial behavior.
>
> One week later, the parents came back eager to tell me about how much Mia had lied between our sessions. Whenever I attempted to elicit from them what was working with Mia, they countered with a barrage of negative responses. Even after using coping and pessimistic questions (Berg & Miller, 1988; Selekman, 1993), the parents continued to remain in a negative mode. I came to a crossroads with the couple; I could pursue the use of imagination and the future with them, externalize the lying problem and its effects, or track the problem sequence in which the lying behavior was embedded and utilize pattern intervention strategies (O'Hanlon, 1987) to break up this pattern.
>
> To help move the couple far away from their present stuck problem-saturated situation with Mia, I decided to give them two tickets to Parentland and inject them into a world of imagination where anything and everything was possible as parents. For the first time, the parents were sporting smiles on their faces and appeared receptive to accepting my invitation to transport them to Parentland. Once the parents began to capture images of parents "laughing," "having fun with their children," and "looking so relaxed," they began to talk about how they wished they could

be "more like this with Mia." I explored with the parents whether they wanted to bring these Parentland ways of being into their own situation with Mia. I had them visualize how Mia would respond to them when they were "laughing" more, "having fun" together, and being much more "relaxed" around her. Both parents described images of seeing a "happier" Mia, wanting to "spend time" with them "playing a game together," and much more "calm in the house." I prescribed for the couple to experiment with these new Parentland positive behaviors for 1 week.

The couple came in for our third session reporting several important changes. Mia was "not caught in a lie once," they reported feeling "much more relaxed," and they "went to an amusement park as a family," an activity that they had not done together for years. The parents also discovered that being less reactive and more patient, and "trying to have fun" as parents were making a difference. I saw the couple two more times, with longer time intervals between visits as a vote of confidence to them. I never had to see Mia, for the parents successfully resolved the lying problem by changing their dance steps.

INVITATION FOR CURIOSITY: ENTER THE REFLECTING TEAM

With some *same* or *worse* category families, we can become quite stuck therapeutically. The reflecting team (Andersen, 1991, 1995) consultation method can provide the therapist and the family with the opportunity to discover alternative views or explanations of the problem story and the events that transpired in the interviewing process. Midway through the session, after the consultation team has given their reflections, the experience can open up space for the family and the therapist to view themselves, their actions, and their relationships differently. The reflecting team can help the family and the therapist move away from viewing the problem story in one particular way. They model for the family many possible explanations for the problem, with no one view being any more "correct" than others (Andersen, 1991). The reflecting team experience also teaches the family that their problem story is not carved in stone or static but in constant evolutionary flux. The family members learn that the tales they tell about the problem are fictionalized accounts (Schafer, 1980) and that they play an active role in their own storymaking. Finally, the reflections by the team are intended to introduce "news of a difference" and to be liberating, not to be corrective or prescriptive (Andersen, 1991, 1995).

Guidelines for the Reflecting Process

The reflecting team format can be conducted in a variety of ways. If a clinic or agency has a one-way mirror or a closed-circuit TV hook-up, midway through the session the interviewing therapist and the family can switch rooms with the consultation team and they can listen quietly to the team's conversation about the problem story and what was discussed earlier in the session. After the team's 6 to 8-minute conversation, the therapist and the family switch rooms again and the family is invited to respond to the team's reflections. Some families wish to have the team in the therapy room, and my colleagues and I honor their request. Another useful reflecting team format is to have a colleague in the therapy room sitting close to the interviewing therapist and the family in the observing position, and midway through the session the therapists have their reflection in front of the family. The family then has an opportunity to reflect on the therapists' conversation. When reflecting, therapists should consider the following rules of thumb:

1. Begin reflections with such qualifiers as "I wonder if . . . "; "Could it be . . . ?"; "What struck me . . . "; "Sometimes . . . " (Reflections need to be presented with a "suspension of disbelief"; Spence, 1982.)

2. Don't bombard the family with too many ideas.

3. Avoid pushing for team consensus with ideas.

4. Keep reflections from becoming long monologues; they should be short and to the point.

5. Avoid pathologizing language or negative explanations that may be interpreted as blaming by family members.

6. Be careful not to make excessive use of positive relabeling, for family members may think you are being sarcastic or trying to talk them out of their problems.

7. Include the interviewing therapist as part of the themes or events on which you are reflecting.

8. Be curious about the missing pieces of the family puzzle, including potential family secrets or the "not yet said" (Ander-

son & Goolishian, 1988b), which you can carefully wonder out loud about with the team.

9. Keep reflections from being too similar or too far removed from how the family views their problem story.

The major strength of the reflecting team method is that it creates a learning climate that celebrates differences, which increases the likelihood for new ideas and meanings to be internalized by family members. A good team reflection can have a liberating effect for the stuck interviewing therapist, helping him or her get out of treatment impasses, gain access to fresh ideas, and discover more effective ways to cooperate with family members. With more challenging family cases, the reflecting team method can be the therapeutic pathway of maximum advantage.

Case Example

Ten-year-old Brian was brought for therapy for "stealing," "bedwetting," "doing poorly in school" gradewise, and constantly testing his parents' limits. He frequently stole toys from his 12-year-old brother's bedroom and teased his 7-year-old sister. After three highly unproductive sessions with this family, I recruited one of my colleagues to team this case with me. Up to this point, I had been unsuccessful at negotiating solvable problems and goals with the parents; the family continued to blame Brian for "all the stress" and "problems" in their family, and Brian's presenting problems got worse. The parents failed to follow through with the assigned therapeutic tasks and Brian would not speak to me at all. In our fourth family session, my colleague Ginger, who was in the room with us in the observing position, offered the following provocative reflection:

> I wonder if Brian ever feels like he lives in a sewer. . . . I had this crazy image that flashed in my mind of Brian's standing at the bottom of a sewer looking up at the beam of light that was shining in his face from the slightly pushed open sewer lid at street level . . . he was patiently waiting for something to happen. . . .

I responded to Ginger's sewer metaphor with a question: "Could it be that Brian was hoping that someone would throw him down a rope or hand him a ladder?" Ginger replied, "Perhaps one or the other." Because I was not sure how well the family would take to Ginger's highly provocative reflection, and I did not want to come across as too allied with her thoughts, I presented the following different perspective on the problem story: "I wonder if Brian is trying to steal back time with his parents . . . this happens sometimes with middle children." When the family was invited to reflect on our reflections, surprisingly both parents found these ideas to be quite newsworthy to them, particularly Ginger's sewer metaphor. The father was so struck by the metaphor that he asked Brian whether he felt like he lived in a sewer. For the first time in therapy, Brian asserted himself and responded to his father with a firm "yes!" He further added, "I feel sometimes like you are trying to flush me down the toilet." Both parents were quite alarmed and concerned that Brian was feeling this way and explored with him what they could do to make him "feel more wanted" and "happier." From this point on, therapy took a productive course. Brian was able to talk about how his siblings monopolized his parents' "attention," which spoke to my reflection along these lines.

I met with the family four more times before concluding therapy. If it were not for the use of the reflecting team format, I would have remained totally stuck with this family, or eventually they would have fired me.

WU WEI: THE PATHWAY OF NONDOING

Lao-tzu's answer to social and human chaos was the doctrine of "inaction," or, in Chinese, *wu wei*. He believed that in human relationships, force defeats itself. Every action produces a reaction, every challenge a response (cited in Barrett, 1993). It was Lao-tzu's contention that *wu wei* was the only means to achieve true success; sooner or later planned intervention would result in failure. He wrote: "Do nondoing, strive for nonstriving, regard the small as important, make much of little" (cited in Barrett, 1993, pp. 29–30). The main strength in the *wu wei* doctrine is that it conveys an attitude that makes all doing both possible and effective.

Nondoing can occur within action as well as in stillness. According to Kabat-Zinn (1994), "The inward stillness of the doer merges with the outward activity to such an extent that the action does itself. There is no exertion of the will, no small-minded 'I,' 'me,' or 'mine' to lay claim to a result, yet nothing is left undone" (p. 40). It takes a great deal of effort and energy to cultivate nondoing.

In the therapeutic arena, practicing nondoing or *wu wei* can help therapists let go of the need to find the "right" questions to ask families in the interviewing process or allow themselves to be distracted by intrusive thoughts regarding the types of therapeutic tasks that would "best" fit a particular family's presenting problems and treatment goal. Sometimes we get so caught up in the family's past problem-saturated story or are so overly focused on co-creating desirable future realities with our clients that we lose touch with the here and now. Staying close to our clients in the present moment is what Buddhists refer to as *mindfulness*. Mindfulness helps foster greater awareness, clarity, and acceptance of the family's present-moment reality (Kabat-Zinn, 1994). Practicing both *wu wei* and mindfulness can be particularly useful with stuck *same-* or *worse*-type families, with which being highly active therapeutically by assigning both in- and out-of-session tasks and being too outcome-focused in the interviewing process have failed to produce any changes with the identified child client and his or her family. By abandoning all our previous unhelpful ideas about trying to get somewhere with or make something happen therapeutically with a particular family, we may accomplish more and be more effective at helping them in the long run.

Rinpoche (1993) recommends another important Buddhist thought-training practice which consists of viewing problems and difficult situations as a benefit to us, in that they make our minds happy. Rinpoche states:

> Whenever a problem arises, be happy by recognizing it as beneficial, by seeing that it supports the generation of the path to enlightenment within your mind. Rejoice each time you meet an obstacle. Immediately think: "This appears to be an obstacle, but actually it is not an obstacle for me. Enjoy it; be happy." (1993, pp. 40–41)

Accepting the problems and impasses we encounter in our client's difficult case situations, rather than allowing ourselves to worry about being therapeutically stuck and ineffective, can make a big difference in transforming our minds and opening up space for possibilities.

Case Example

Charlotte brought her three children—11-year-old Julie, 10-year-old Warren, and 8-year-old Mary Lou—in for treatment to help them better cope with their "alcoholic father." All three children were experiencing problems with anxiety, depression, and somatic complaints, which Charlotte felt were all caused by their "father's disease." The father, Robert, had refused to come for counseling with his family. According to Charlotte, Robert had already experienced "two inpatient treatment failures for alcoholism" because he "refused to go to AA [Alcoholics Anonymous] meetings" and attend his "outpatient counseling sessions." Julie's grades were "slipping" in school, she was experiencing "headaches," and she looked very depressed in our first family session. Warren presented himself as very engaging and playful but "suffering from chronic stomachaches." Mary Lou presented herself as extremely shy and said very little in the session. Charlotte had been receiving "codependency" treatment for 2 years and was actively involved in her local Al-Anon support group. I asked the family both the miracle (de Shazer, 1988) and imaginary wand questions, but the children had a very hard time contributing anything that would indicate an ideal miracle or a wished outcome picture for them. None of the children mentioned anything about their father either when I asked them about what they viewed as the problem or after asking these two questions.

Charlotte, on the other hand, had no problem reeling off miracles about how the children would be symptom-free, "happier," "doing better in school," and "talking about their thoughts and feelings about having an alcoholic father." It was interesting to note that the children tuned out their mother when she brought up their father's name. At this point in the session, because goal setting proved to be impossible, I divided up the remaining times and met alone with Charlotte to explore her attempted solutions and then with the children to try an art therapy task.

Charlotte had tried to do a variety of things to help her children get "more in touch" with their "feelings," such as taking them to a few Ala-Tot meetings, "including them" in the past in her "counseling sessions" when she had been working on her own "codependency problem," and pulling each child aside and asking them "how they felt about having an alcoholic father." In an attempt to better enter Charlotte's 12-Step recovery world, I explored with her whether she might be inadvertently "enabling" her children not to talk about their father's "disease" by putting pressure on them to do so. I recommended that she experiment for a week of "detaching with love" from "asking them about how they feel about" their father. Charlotte found this suggestion intriguing and could see how her attempted solution of trying to make them talk about their feelings was "backfiring" and making matters worse. We also decided that I would try to engage Robert and see him individually for a session.

As a way to better join with the children and do things differently, I had each one draw a family portrait. When they completed their drawings, I brought Charlotte into the room and invited each child to tell his or her story about the art products. Both Julie and Warren left their father out of their pictures. When Charlotte asked them about this, we got such responses as: "I don't know" and "He's not here." Mary Lou included her father in her picture, standing right next to the rest of the family. Again, Charlotte pushed for explanations and feelings and Mary Lou said, "I want Daddy with us." Mary Lou was the closest to her father of all of the siblings. We scheduled another appointment for 1 week later.

Robert failed to come to our scheduled individual session. Instead, he showed up at our next family session. His excuse for not coming to the individual session was that he had to "work late" and "forgot" to call to cancel. Robert's presence in the family session had a silencing effect on all family members. He also smelled of alcohol. When I met alone with Charlotte and Robert, the two started to argue and Charlotte disclosed for the first time that after 15 years of marriage, she planned to pursue a "divorce."

Because it proved to be counterproductive to see the couple together, I saw them separately. Robert spent most of his time devaluing all the therapists and hospital treatment experiences with which he had been involved. He also blamed his wife for their "marital problems." Robert made it very clear to me that he would not come back, because I "could not help" him. Charlotte shared with me during our individual session time together that she was quite angry at Robert for coming to the session intoxicated and that she had already contacted an attorney about filing for a divorce. As there was very little session time left to meet with the children, we decided to devote the majority of the next session to the children.

Upon reflecting on my therapeutic activity with this family in the first two sessions, it was clear that in some ways I was replicating the mother's dances with the children. I, too, was pushing the children to talk about their thoughts and feelings about their father and being superresponsible around them by trying to find the "right" question to ask them or the "right" therapeutic task that would stabilize their symptoms. I was not in the present moment with Charlotte's family, my mind was too preoccupied with the following thoughts:

"What am I going to do that will work with this family?"
"We don't have a small realistic treatment goal?"
"How am I going to be able to change all of the multiple symptom-bearers in this family?"

It was clear that I needed to do something dramatically different as a therapist to get unstuck and break my unhelpful patterns of relating to the family, including thoughts that were too focused on outcome.

When I met with the family for the third time, I made a number of therapeutic adjustments. First and foremost, I began to practice *wu wei* and mindfulness while in process with the family. Instead of being highly active and structuring the session, I followed each family member's lead in terms of what he or she wanted to talk about or how he or she wanted to use the session time. I used more open-ended conversational questions (Anderson & Goolishian, 1988a, 1988b), which gave family members much more room to tell their stories unedited by me.

I ended up seeing Charlotte's family 10 more times over a year. By practicing *wu wei* and mindfulness and taking each family member as he or she was, I was successful in stabilizing the children's symptoms and empowering Charlotte to lead her family as a single parent in a more positive and preferred direction. Robert dropped out of treatment after our first encounter together. Charlotte had Robert legally removed from their home. Charlotte also carried through with divorce. The most dramatic change with the children was their ability to open up spontaneously about their sad and angry feelings toward the father, both in conversation and when processing their art products. As a postscript, I received a call from Charlotte 2 years later telling me that she was remarried and her children were doing great emotionally, socially, and academically.

THE JOYS OF THERAPEUTIC FAILURE

Most well-known family therapy gurus and therapists in general rarely discuss their treatment failures. I have yet to go to a workshop and experience the family therapy guru showing videotaped examples of or discussing his or her case failures. For a number of reasons (pride, to name one), most of us have a tendency to sweep our therapeutic blunders under the carpet and to view failure as a bad thing. However, it is my contention that we should joyously embrace our therapeutic blunders and failures and view them as some of our best teachers. Failures provide us with valuable wisdom and are an integral part of the creative problem-solving process. Failures can teach us to stop thinking that we are privileged experts, to bring back curiosity to help keep our minds dynamic, to stop trying to emulate our gurus but be ourselves and develop our own unique therapeutic styles, to be more therapeutically flexible, to avoid falling into the trap of one-size-fits-all therapy complacency, and to expand our horizons and learn about new therapy approaches and techniques that we can add to our therapeutic repertoire. Finally, therapy failures can help us grow personally and professionally.

Firing Yourself

With some child cases, no matter what the therapist does or doesn't do, he or she fails to make a difference in resolving the child's and family's presenting problems. One therapeutic strategy that is a good last-ditch intervention when everything else has failed is for therapists to fire themselves. I tell the family that I have obviously missed the boat with them in terms of understanding and helping them resolve their problems. I further add that they should have a new therapist with fresh ideas who could be more helpful to them. I then offer to introduce them to one of my colleagues who will take over their case. Typically what happens with this intervention is that the parents in particular become more realistic in their expectations of the therapist and, for the first time in treatment, a cooperative working relationship begins to develop. Also, families hate to let go of a therapist because they don't want to have to tell their long, problem-saturated story all over again to a new therapist. This intervention is particularly effective with parents who refuse to budge from their position of viewing the therapist as the expert who will "fix" their child and for parents who repeatedly fail to follow through with assigned therapeutic tasks and fail to see how their rigid beliefs and unhelpful attempted solutions maintain the child's problems.

In the case example that follows, the biological parents and the stepmother fit all the criterion described for utilizing this therapeutic strategy. However, they beat me to the punch and fired me first. I have often wondered whether, if I had fired myself, the outcome with this family would have been different.

Trapped in a Postdivorce Black Hole

Danny, 10 years old, was brought for therapy by his stepmother Louise for "low self-esteem," "depression," and great difficulty "expressing his thoughts and feelings." Danny's parents had been "divorced for 3 years." His mother, Rachel, was granted "legal custody." The father, Richard, had Danny during the "summer months." It was clear to me in the very first session that there was bad blood between Louise and Rachel. Louise spent the early part of the first session bad-mouthing Rachel and pointing out how Richard could provide a "better home" for Danny. Because it seemed countertherapeutic to have Danny listen to Louise's verbally bashing his mother, I had him sit out in the waiting room.

While meeting alone with Louise, she continued to put down Rachel. She also wanted me to know that Rachel had gone out of her way legally to stretch out the divorce process as a way to further frustrate Richard. I found myself feeling both frustrated and tired of listening to Louise's blaming. When I inquired about Richard's availability, Louise had all kind of excuses for why Richard could not come for the first few sessions. Surprisingly, Louise ended up apologizing for spending so much time bad-mouthing Rachel and admitted that she should not do this in front of Danny. I stressed the importance of divorced parents and stepparents working together around the children and how crucial this is in helping the children with the postdivorce adjustment process. Louise agreed with me and was receptive to my idea having some joint sessions with Rachel. Her goal was for Danny to be "better able to open" up about the divorce situation.

When I met with Danny alone, he had his head down and looked very sad. I asked Danny how I could be most helpful to him. Danny took a risk with me and told me that he didn't like Louise because she was "trying to replace my mom." Danny also described Louise as being "mean" to his "mother on the telephone" and when she "picks" him "up." I asked Danny if he thought it might be helpful for him to confront Louise about these things in one of our future sessions. Although Danny thought it was a good idea, he told me that he was "scared" that his "dad would get mad." I complimented him on his courage to share his concerns with me. Danny liked the idea of involving his mom in family sessions. I found out from Danny that his father had been "away a lot on business trips" during most of his summer stay.

In my second session with Danny and Louise, Louise felt "it would be best" that I devoted the bulk of the "session time to her stepson" because she had to run some errands and she felt he would probably "open up more" to me without her "in the room." Before Louise left, I met with her briefly alone to see whether I could negotiate a solvable treatment goal. I explored with Louise what the signs of Danny's being "more open with his feelings" would look like and how she would be able to tell that the problem was really solved. Unfortunately, all Louise could give me was more vagueness about what her ideal outcome picture would look like. However, she did make it clear to me that it was Richard's and her hope in the future that Danny would "live with" them when "he gets older." After Louise left the room, I became suspicious that bringing Danny to see me was part of their possible future plan to build a legal case to win custody of him, especially to get me in their corner so that I would say it was in the best interest of the child, for psychological reasons, to live with them.

Danny was in better spirits this session, and seemed happier. I asked him which home he felt most comfortable living in. Danny voiced a strong desire to remain in his mother's home. He shared with me that he was upset that his dad was "away" so much.

My third and fourth sessions were with Danny and Rachel. It was easy to warm up to Rachel. She was a hardworking career woman and appeared very loving and concerned about Danny's well-being. When I met alone with her in both sessions, she disclosed to me how she was having a hard time dealing with Louise, more so than Richard.

One week after this last session with Rachel and Danny, Louise called me on the telephone and chewed me out. She claimed that I was "not very professional taking Rachel's side" and that I wasn't "good for Danny" either. Whenever I tried to get in a word, Louise continued to devalue me and would not listen. Eventually, she hung up on me. Whenever I called Louise, she would hang up on me, so no further sessions could be scheduled. I notified Rachel about what had happened and she said, "I'm not surprised. . . . Louise is into power plays."

Case Analysis

In analyzing this case and thinking about what I would have done differently if I had the opportunity to turn back the clock, I probably would have kept things simple and worked only with Louise, Richard, and Danny. I should have been more aggressive in trying to engage

Richard. There was so much bad blood between Louise, Richard, and Rachel that my actively involving Rachel was probably perceived as a threat. I felt that I was on the right track in my individual work with Danny. There is a part of me that still believes that the real reason I was fired by Louise was my unwillingness to take her side against Rachel and fit into their possible future plans to try to gain legal custody of Danny. As with most divorcing or postdivorce family cases, it is easy for the therapist to lose his or her therapeutic maneuverability and get trapped. Once trapped in secrets or taking sides, the therapist can get swallowed up by the postdivorce black hole and be powerless to help move the family into new realities. This was the case with Danny's family. However, I gained some important therapeutic wisdom from Danny's case, such as encouraging family members in the divorce process or in postdivorce situations to communicate their feelings, thoughts, and conflicts directly with one another rather than with me alone. It also might have been advantageous to use a reflecting team format with this family. I have found in the past that a reflecting team format is most useful with challenging divorcing and postdivorce family cases.

The next treatment failure case could have fit nicely in the "your worst nightmare" category. Not only were both the mother and daughter oppressed by chronic health problems and psychosocial stressors, but the twosome were socially isolated and struggling to get by financially. I also discovered from the mother, Tamara, that I was the seventh therapist she had taken her 8-year-old daughter, Yolanda, to see. Tamara referred to Yolanda as being "a bad seed."

"She's Just a Bad Seed"

Tamara, a 45-year-old African American woman, brought Yolanda in to see me at the request of Yolanda's school social worker because of Yolanda's "ADHD condition," oppositional behavior, and "not listening" to her teacher and other school staff. Yolanda was on Ritalin and had been placed in a behavior disorder school program. Tamara was also concerned about Yolanda's lack of self-management in "taking care of her diabetes" problem. Yolanda would steal candy from stores and eat just enough to warrant a trip to her pediatrician's office. While Tamara was reeling off all Yolanda's problems, Yolanda started to play with my desk computer. Tamara screamed at Yolanda and then turned to me and said: "You see what I mean, she's just a bad seed!" Tamara grabbed Yolanda and made her sit in a chair right next to her. Tamara went on to tell me that she wished she could "send Yolanda down South" to her "mother's to live," but her concern was that all the stress involved in raising Yolanda "would kill" her mother.

Yolanda was not the only one with multiple individual problems. Tamara had "leukemia" and "severe arthritis" in her legs, was on disability because of her debilitating health problems, and was on Prozac for depression. She frequently had to see her primary care physician for her health problems. Tamara saw her psychiatrist for medication management every 3 months.

After giving Tamara plenty of room to tell her long, problem-saturated story, taking a developmental history on Yolanda, and finding out how the family felt about working with a white therapist, I asked them both the miracle (de Shazer, 1988) and imaginary wand questions. Tamara made it quite clear to me that she could not envision any miracles happening with either her or Yolanda. Yolanda was totally silent. Even after shifting gears and asking Tamara both coping and pessimistic questions (Berg & Miller, 1992; Selekman, 1993), she continued to be pessimistic and could not identify any exceptions that had occurred with Yolanda. Tamara also shared with me that she had no problem working with a white therapist; her former therapists, medical doctors, and psychiatrist had all been white. At this point in the session, I had Yolanda go out to the waiting room and I met alone with Tamara to see whether I could negotiate solvable problems and goals with her and find out what her attempted solutions had been in trying to resolve her daughter's behavioral problems.

Tamara indicated to me that she was feeling emotionally and physically drained by her individual problems and Yolanda's difficulties. Tamara could not identify any one behavior that she wanted me to work on changing with Yolanda. Her expectations of me were monolithic, "Could you change her personality . . . I mean . . . maybe if you could find out what's going on in her mind? . . . " I shared with her that we needed to go for a smaller change and focus on behaviors versus trying to figure out "why." This discussion went nowhere. I then explored Tamara's attempted solutions, which were "yelling" a lot, "taking toys away," "not letting her go to play," praying a lot, and occasionally giving her "whippings" (spanking her on the buttocks). When I asked Tamara about her past treatment experiences, she quickly pointed out that the psychologists' and social workers' "behavioral management programs did not work on Yolanda." I then asked her if she had any ideas for me about what I could do differently as a therapist that might make a difference for her and Yolanda. Tamara responded, "I don't know." She also refused to give me written consent to collaborate with the school staff and her psychiatrist. Tamara felt that the past therapists' involvement with the school staff had made matters worse by leading to Yolanda's placement in the behavior disorder program and being scapegoated. She would not tell me why I could not talk with her psychiatrist. Finally, Tamara made it clear to me that she wanted me to do "individual therapy" with Yolanda.

Because Tamara was relating to me more like a complainant than a customer, I was tempted to give her an observation task, but intuitively I felt that she would probably not follow through with this task because she believed strongly that Yolanda was the problem. I also thought that this was a "disconnected family" (Selekman, 1993) situation—in that a change in either one of these family members would not trigger a change in the other. Somehow I felt that I needed to work with them separately, establish separate goals, and eventually have each of them do things differently around one another. I decided to err on the side of caution with Tamara and not give her a task. I did, however, give her a few compliments about being committed as a parent and being resilient. I also gave her information about some community-based support groups for parents.

My individual session time with Yolanda also proved to be highly unproductive. Yolanda refused to talk to me and would not engage in either a board game or an art task.

Sessions two through six ended up being replays of this initial family interview. It reminded me of the movie *Groundhog Day*, with the actor Bill Murray, who repeatedly woke up and experienced the same day over and over again. As an attempt to try to do something differently, I introduced the idea of using a reflecting team format, but Tamara found it too intrusive to have "strangers watch our sessions." I was still unable to get Tamara to give me written consent to collaborate with the school or her psychiatrist. In session two, I gave Tamara the Do Something Different task (de Shazer, 1985), but she did not follow through with it. I was never able to join well enough with Yolanda for her to open up with me about how I could be helpful to her. The family dropped out of treatment after our sixth session. After a few months had passed and Tamara failed to return my phone calls or respond to my letters, I decided to close their case.

Case Analysis

In analyzing this case, there are two things I would have done differently with this family if I had the opportunity to work with them again.

First, I was stuck doing more of the same (Watzlawick et al., 1974) with the mother, putting too much pressure on her to be part of the solution-construction process and trying to secure written consent to collaborate with the school and her psychiatrist. Second, I should have accepted Tamara's belief that Yolanda was the problem and then greatly exaggerated the severity of her daughter's problems as an attempt to draw Tamara in more and to collaborate with her about what she could do to help prevent the situation from getting worse. Another strategy I could have pursued with Yolanda and her mother would have been to externalize one of Yolanda's chronic presenting problems. Because the school had made the referral, I felt it was critical to collaborate with them and also to try to resolve the conflicts between school personnel, Tamara, and Yolanda. I also thought it would be useful to collaborate with Tamara's psychiatrist so that we were supporting what each other was doing therapeutically with Tamara.

I could recall many times throughout the course of therapy, when I was feeling stuck in sessions, that I had wished that Scottie from the TV show *Star Trek* would beam me up to the Starship Enterprise. However, this case taught me a lot of important lessons—such as that sometimes being too technique-oriented or outcome-focused with certain families can keep the problems intact or make things worse. This case also reminded me of the importance of observing ourselves in relationship to our clients. If I had been a better self-observer with this family, I might have been better able to stop myself from doing more of the same (Watzlawick et al., 1974). Finally, cases like Tamara's remind us that when we are working harder than our clients, therapeutic changes are highly unlikely to happen.

CONCLUSION

In this chapter, I have presented several different therapeutic pathways for therapists to pursue when working with "impossible" cases. I have also stressed the importance of viewing intractable client problems, therapeutic impasses, and treatment failures as our best teachers. They remind us to be therapeutically flexible and that professional knowledge and wisdom is always on the way.

CHAPTER 9

Helping Children and Their Families Succeed in a Managed Care World

Doing is knowing, which leads to a new client story.
                                                    –STEVE DE SHAZER

INTRODUCTION:
THE WORLD OF MANAGED HEALTH CARE

For decades, mental health professionals had the freedom to keep children in treatment for as long as they deemed necessary. Children were typically seen individually for play therapy, while the parents were often seen separately by another therapist, or sometimes occasionally by the same therapist who was treating the child. In the past, it was not uncommon for child therapists to see their young clients until their parents' indemnity health plan benefit was exhausted for the calendar year. More recently, however, major insurance companies and large corporations have initiated a major crusade to reduce the exorbitant health care costs of their subscribers and employers, respectively. According to Browning (1996), health care costs rose 193% between 1983 and 1993. Hence, managed care companies have been created to ensure that insurees receive efficient and cost-effective quality treatment. General Motors provides one good example of how a major corporation's employee health care costs got out of control. In 1994, General Motors spent more money on health care costs for its employees than on the sheet metal it purchased to build their cars (Woods, 1995)! In my own clinical practice with children and their families, I can think of numerous cases where children were misdiagnosed, were wrongly institutionalized, and received ineffective treatments that further compounded and exacerbated their problem situations.

Although managed care has been around for more than two decades, many therapists view managed care companies as the enemy. Common complaints are that managed care companies are intrusive and only invested in cutting costs and making a profit, and the case managers providing the telephone case reviews are incompetent and clinically inexperienced. In response to these complaints, factions of private practitioners and other mental health professionals do battle with managed care and lobby for governmental regulation of these companies in an effort to scrutinize their management of cases and other activities. Having worked for a major managed care company for 5 years, I have no doubt that sometimes cases fall between the cracks and are mismanaged and that contracted network providers are treated badly by the utilization review team. To my knowledge, no managed care company exists that has a flawless care management delivery system. Some managed care companies are more solid and enjoy better reputations than others. Some successful private practitioners with glowing reputations in their respective communities may be able to continue to thrive on fee-for-service business and bypass managed care systems. However, the world of private practice is becoming increasingly competitive and fee-for-service business may start to dry up. The stalwart private practitioners will then be forced to explore other markets for business. By the year 2000, many predict that indemnity health insurance plans will be obsolete. In 1996, 124.7 million people were enrolled in managed behavioral health programs (Oss & Stair, 1996). As enrollments are on the rise, anti-managed care and long-term-oriented therapists may eventually have to revisit the idea of contracting with managed care companies as their primary source of business.

GUIDELINES FOR EMPOWERING FAMILIES TO SUCCEED IN THEIR MANAGED CARE TREATMENT EXPERIENCES

Because many clinicians today, by choice or by administrative mandate, work with managed care companies, it is crucial to help parents understand and learn how to work with the managed care treatment delivery system in order to receive the most optimal care for their children. Six practical guidelines will aid therapists in their communications with case managers, help increase the number of referrals they receive, and empower children and their families so they will succeed in their managed care treatment experiences.

Educate Families about Managed Care

Therapists serving on managed care company provider networks need to be familiar with the business aspects and treatment guidelines of each managed care company with which they are contracted. All managed care companies have manuals spelling out levels-of-care treatment guidelines for Axis I DSM-IV diagnoses, as well as exclusionary diagnoses that are not covered by the insurance plan. It is crucial that families be educated on the basic nuts and bolts of managed care, including the importance of medical necessity for authorizing visits; emphasis on symptom stabilization, not insight or growth; the fact that managed care companies were created for cost-containment purposes and to ensure that clients are given the best necessary treatment within the limitations of their health plan; an explanation of the role of the case manager in the treatment process; and the fact that the case manager serves as an advocate for the client in securing authorization for therapy when necessary.

Educating families early in therapy about what to expect in a managed-care-driven treatment context can greatly help them be more realistic in regard to their treatment expectations and goals. It is also important to share with families that they will serve as collaborators in the treatment process, not only that their goals will drive the treatment but that they will regularly be given homework assignments between visits to help them achieve their goals rapidly. Once therapy sessions have been authorized, part of the goal-setting process should be to ask clients, "We have six sessions to work with. What do you want to work on changing first?" Experience has taught me, as a case manager and contracted network provider, that telling families they have a limited number of sessions to work with helps mobilize their strengths and resources and heighten their motivation levels to make something happen quickly.

Ask Families about Pretreatment Changes

Research indicates that clients often take some important steps toward resolving their presenting problems between the time of their telephone call to a clinic or agency and their first scheduled appointment (Allgood, Parham, Salts, & Smith, 1995; Bloom, 1981; Howard, Kopta, Krause, & Orlinsky, 1986; Johnson & Nelson, 1996; Selekman, 1993; Talmon, 1990, 1993; Weiner-Davis, de Shazer, & Gingerich, 1987). Howard et al. (1986) found in their study that 15% of the clients reported "feeling better" and showed measurable improvement before attending their first session. Weiner-Davis et al. (1987) and Talmon (1990) report even better results in their studies. Some of the researchers attribute clients' pretreatment changes to "spontaneous remission," which can occur through the process of simply making an appointment. This initial telephone call lowers some clients' distress levels based on the fact that they will soon receive help. In their study, Johnson and Nelson (1996) found that 79% of their clients who reported pretreatment changes indicated that the reported changes continued well after three therapy sessions. Selekman (1993) and Weiner-Davis et al. (1987) attribute their clients' pretreatment changes to the fact that all parents and their children have the strengths and resources to change. Therefore, therapists' expertise should be in eliciting their client's expertise. In an initial family assessment session, the therapist should ask families the following questions:

> "Many times between the time of the phone call to our clinic and the first session clients take some important steps toward improving their situation. What have each of you noticed that is different or better with your situation?"
>
> "Wow! How did you get that to happen?"
>
> "Is that different for your son or daughter to do that?"
>
> "Is your situation better enough in that area now?"
>
> "What else is better?"
>
> "How will I know that you are confident enough for us to stop?"

While gathering information about each reported pretreatment change, the therapist should play detective and elicit details from family members about what they are doing that increases the likelihood of these solution patterns of behavior and thinking occurring (de Shazer & White, 1996). Collaboratively, the therapist and the family can attempt to co-construct a solution out of these pretreatment building blocks for change.

As a way to help families become more aware of their unique strengths and innate problem-solving and coping capacities, Selekman (1993) and Talmon (1990) have intake workers and assigned therapists give families a task assignment prior to coming in for their first family assessment sessions. A parent would be given the following assignment:

> In order for [_____therapist's name_____] to learn what you and your family's strengths and goals are, we would like you to notice what's

happening in your relationship with [____the identified client____]
and in your family that you would like to continue to have happen.
Please write what you observed down and bring your list with you
when you come for your first appointment.

Not only has this pretreatment assignment empowered families to
resolve their own difficulties, but it can greatly reduce lengths of stay
in treatment, which is quite appealing to managed care companies. This
pretreatment task assignment strategy can also be a useful solution for
agencies and clinics faced with horrendous waiting-list problems. If we
see clients for shorter durations as a result of capitalizing on their
pretreatment changes, we can see more clients and quickly resolve the
waiting-list problem.

Speak the Language of Change with Families and Case Managers

Throughout the course of treatment, it is most advantageous for
therapists to speak the language of change with their clients and case
managers. By the language of change I mean conveying, as early as
possible, that change will happen with their situations and it is only a
matter of when. Having a family describe in great detail their ideal
outcome picture once their problems are solved—the *who, what, when,*
and *how* of goal attainment—as well as their past successes, can empower them and raise their expectation level for change. De Shazer
and his colleagues at the Brief Therapy Center in Milwaukee, Wisconsin, have provided some empirical support for the relationship between
therapists' use of "solution talk" with their clients and positive treatment outcomes (de Shazer, 1994; Gingerich et al., 1988).

When communicating with case managers, therapists should utilize solution talk, such as reporting family members' strengths, past
successes and pretreatment changes, family goals that are realistic and
behavioral, while conveying optimism and confidence in their ability
to help the family achieve their goals. There is no question that case
managers who receive a report from a provider that is outcome-ori-
ented and based on client strengths will expect this provider to be more
likely to help his or her clients successfully achieve their goals. Once
the provider establishes a solid track record, the likelihood of the
provider's receiving a fairly steady stream of referrals increases.

In treatment update reports, therapists need to clearly articulate
the following to case managers: how well the family's presenting
symptoms are stabilizing, whether the family has achieved their goals,

and a good rationale for the need for additional visits, particularly for consolidating gains or to further stabilize the presenting symptoms. Case managers also favor providers who schedule longer time intervals between visits, particularly as a vote of confidence when clients are progressing.

Case Managers and Network Providers Share Problem System Membership

Once a contracted provider accepts a referral from a case manager, he or she become part of the problem system. In fact, all individuals involved in identifying the child's problems and trying to solve them comprise the problem system membership (Anderson & Goolishian, 1988b; Selekman, 1993). In a managed care treatment context, the problem system may include the following individuals: the provider, the case manager, the case manager's supervisor, the utilization management team, possibly an involved employee assistance program counselor from one parent's job, the child, his or her family, and possibly school personnel and the family's primary care physician. Throughout the family treatment process, the provider needs to be sensitive to the fact that all these individuals can play an active role in the maintenance of the family problems, as well as being a part of the solution.

As early as possible in the referral process, the network provider needs to foster a cooperative and collaborative relationship with the assigned case manager. What is most important to remember is that each case manager we work with will have a unique way of cooperating with us. For example, some case managers want to be actively involved in the client treatment planning process, while others defer to the provider's clinical judgment (Browning, 1996). Ideally, we should try to cooperate with the unique cooperative styles of each case manager from whom we receive referrals. Relationship skills such as humor, warmth, empathy, and being flexible are important ingredients for helping foster a collaborative relationship with case managers. Network providers need to be team players and to view case managers as allies rather than the enemy. They need to keep the lines of communication open with case managers, alerting them promptly to budding crises, the need for psychiatric backup, and changes in the treatment plan. When stuck with a challenging case, the case manager should be used as a consultant. Never assume that the case manager is not clinically knowledgeable or competent.

We need to be sensitive and respectful of the arduous task, stressful job, and responsibilities of case managers. On a daily basis, they have to juggle cost containment for the managed care company and keeping the client, the parent, the insurance company, and network providers satisfied with how the care management process is being conducted, as well as ensuring that the best necessary treatment is being provided within the scope of the client's benefits. Besides being empathetic with case managers when they are having rough days, providers need to be flexible and open to compromising with the number of therapy visits for which they are requesting authorization during the treatment process. As long as the provider makes a strong case for medical necessity and for the need for more visits to address a recent new development or crisis in the client's life, the case manager should be more than willing to authorize additional visits.

The more effort the provider puts into cultivating solid working relationships with case managers, the more likely case managers are to send referrals. Thus, the case manager becomes part of the solution on two levels, authorizing enough visits to help the client succeed in treatment and providing the therapist with more business to help his or her practice grow.

Negotiate Realistic Treatment Plans and Goals with Families

One study conducted by a large managed care company to assess key characteristics of highly effective providers in its networks found that highly effective therapists were significantly more likely to have been rated by their clients as understanding their problems and as having helped them develop treatment plans to empower them to resolve their problems (Hiatt & Hargrave, 1995). This study was conducted with several thousand clients and contracted network providers. Research of this kind helps support the need for therapists to negotiate realistic treatment plans, that consist of solvable problems, small and realistic behavioral goals, and an efficient therapeutic action plan geared to helping their clients achieve their goals as rapidly as possible.

Therapists can negotiate solvable problems and goals with their clients by asking the following questions:

"How will you know when you don't have to come here anymore?"

"What do you need to see happen here today that will make you feel like this is a good idea?"

"If you were to show me a videotape of this family once your problems were solved, what will we see you doing differently on this video?"

"Let's say you were to drive home from our clinic today and the session we had together proved to be highly successful, what will have changed with your situation?"

"What will be a small sign of progress over the next week that will tell you that you are making headway?"

"How will you know that you are really succeeding with your goal?"

"How confident are you on a scale of 1 to 10, with 10 being totally confident, that we will resolve your son's temper tantrum problem?"

(*To a mother who rated the problem situation to be at a 6*) "Let's say that you and your son return in one week and you proceed to tell me that your son took some steps to get up to a 7. What will you tell me he did?" (Berg & de Shazer, 1993; de Shazer, 1994; O'Hanlon & Weiner-Davis, 1989; Selekman, 1993).

It is helpful to share with families that we are going for small changes that can lead to bigger changes over time. When parents bring their children in to have their "attitude" and "self-esteem" problems "fixed," it is important for the therapist to negotiate these vague difficulties into behavioral terms by asking the following questions:

"When your son has a better attitude, what will he be doing instead?"

"How else will he show you that he has a better attitude?"

"What will be some indicators happening over the next week that will tell you that your daughter has higher self-esteem?"

"What else will she be doing differently that will tell you that her self-esteem is higher?"

Once the family's problems and goals have been negotiated into solvable terms, a therapeutic task to perform between visits can be designed or selected based on family members' unique cooperative response patterns (de Shazer, 1988, 1991, 1994; Selekman, 1993). It is helpful to explain to families that most of their changes will occur outside the office when they successfully follow through with assigned tasks. All tasks designed or selected for family members need to be behavioral and manageable and to fit with the unique cooperative response pattern of each family member. The therapist needs to be clear and concrete when delivering his or her rationale for and description of the mechanics of each task offered. For most families, it can be useful not only to write down their assigned tasks so that they are very clear about what they are expected to do but also to offer them a menu of tasks from which to choose, which can further enhance therapeutic cooperation.

Avoid Setting Up Antagonistic Relationships with Case Managers

The worst professional move a contracted network provider can make is to set up a split between the client and the case manager. We need to view the case manager as an ally, even if we disagree about the number of visits being authorized for our client. It is all right to advocate for the client in a constructive and direct manner with the case manager, but if the provider bypasses this step and complains to the case manager's supervisor, he or she will lose a potential future referral source and quite possibly the business from the other case managers at the managed care company.

Some clients are masters at setting up splits among people and systems in general. It is important first to assess whether this problem needs to be addressed with the client directly. Most case managers are open to collaborating on sticky and challenging cases if the provider is unable to solve impasses with his or her clients. If attempts to constructively resolve a splitting situation between the client and case manager prove to be futile or the provider is gridlocked in a conflictual relationship with a particular case manager, it is the provider's right to consult with the case manager's supervisor.

THE ART OF WRITING BLUE-RIBBON TREATMENT UPDATE REQUESTS

To ensure that families receive enough authorized therapy visits to adequately stabilize the child's symptoms and consolidate family gains, we must clearly indicate the following in our treatment update request forms to managed care companies: the initial treatment goals, treatment interventions and modalities used to help the family achieve their goals, and a good and realistic rationale for the need for authorized additional therapy visits to complete treatment. Once a case manager receives the provider's treatment update request form, he or she will carefully examine the document to make sure the provider has negotiated small, realistic behavioral goals with the family and that the treatment modality being utilized is the most efficient form of therapy for the nature of the child's presenting problem. If the case manager receives a treatment update request from a therapist indicating that he or she is providing mostly individual play therapy with the identified child client to help the child work through his or her unresolved conflict about the parental divorce, and doing very little conjoint family work even with the custodial parent, the case manager may request that another contracted provider or the managed care company's consulting psychiatrist do an independent assessment before any further visits are authorized. The case manager will also carefully read the therapist's rationale for additional therapy visits to make sure it is clear and in line with the initial treatment goals or the new goal negotiated with the clients and that the therapist is not requesting an exorbitant number of visits to complete treatment. Most case managers like to see that the therapist is spacing out the requested visits as a vote of confidence to the clients, using a visit or two to collaborate with involved helping professionals from larger systems, and using the remaining visits to further stabilize the child's symptoms and consolidate family gains. If clinically indicated, the therapist should also mention, in the treatment update request form, the decision to refer the parents to a support group as part of the after-care plans.

Two Examples of Treatment Update Requests

After presenting examples of both a problematic and an accepted treatment update request for additional therapy visits for the same case I provide a comparative analysis of the two update requests. The first example would be red-flagged as problematic by a case manager at any major managed care company. The second example of a treatment update request would be awarded a blue ribbon by most case managers and would lead to the authorization of further visits.

The case presented involved 10-year-old Stephen, diagnosed oppositional defiant, and his parents. The presenting problems were not following parental rules and responding to their limits, swearing at the parents, and testing his teacher's limits in the classroom. Stephen was school-referred by his teacher for chronically mouthing off to her and breaking the classroom rules. The family had been seen by the therapist six times and a treatment update request form for additional visits was mailed to the case manager.

PROBLEMATIC TREATMENT UPDATE REPORT

TREATMENT UPDATE FORM

Name: Stephen Greenway   *Case Number:* 0000
Birth Date: 9-10-86   *Date First Seen:* 10-21-96
SS#: 000-00-0000
Number of Sessions to Date: 6
Diagnosis: 313.81

Client Goals and Treatment Plan: The parents began treatment requesting that I try to find out why Stephen was so angry, swore a lot, and did not follow their rules or his teacher's in her classroom. Although I spent some time teaching the parents some new skills for improving family communications, most of my session time has been devoted to building a trusting relationship with Stephen. Stephen has done a nice job of following my office rules about putting games and art supplies away. He has also opened up to me about how he dislikes when his father "yells loudly" at him. Because Stephen and I are starting to make good headway in treatment, I will continue to see him individually. I will also address the father's "yelling" problem.

Rationale for Additional Sessions: Because it takes time to build a trusting relationship with children, I will need additional visits to do the real therapeutic work with Stephen. To do conjoint family therapy will be far too anxiety-provoking for Stephen. He already is quite anxious about his father's "yelling" all the time. Through the use of play and art therapy techniques, I hope to eventually get at the root of Stephen's impulsivity, anger management difficulties, and oppositional behaviors. Finally, it may also be helpful for me to meet with Stephen's teacher to explore her views about the problem.

Additional Sessions Requested to Complete Treatment: 20

ACCEPTED TREATMENT UPDATE REPORT

TREATMENT UPDATE FORM

Name: Stephen Greenway   *Case Number:* 000
Birthdate: 9-10-86   *Date First Seen:* 10-21-96
SS#: 000-00-0000
Number of Sessions to Date: 6
Diagnosis: 313.81

Client Goals and Treatment Plan: The parents and I began treatment by negotiating the following three goals for Stephen:

1. Increasing compliance with following household rules.
2. Decreasing swearing behavior.
3. Actively collaborating with Stephen's teacher to help decrease disruptive behavior in the classroom.

Stephen and his parents have made considerable headway in all three of these target goal areas. Through the use of Solution-Focused Therapy interventions, the parents are yelling less and positively reinforcing Stephen's prosocial behaviors more, Stephen is more compliant with the parents' rules and swearing less, and Stephen's teacher is reporting marked behavioral improvement in her classroom. The parents are no longer trying to impose unrealistic consequences like taking his computer and TV privileges away for weeks. Stephen also acknowledges that his parents are "being nicer" and "more fair" with him now. I will continue to use an integrative Solution-Focused Therapy approach with the family to consolidate gains and wrap up my involvement with Stephen's teacher.

Rationale for Additional Sessions: Because Stephen and his parents have achieved their goals, I will only need two sessions to consolidate their gains and wrap up my collaborative work with Stephen's teacher. I will space out these visits over the next 2 months as a vote of confidence to the family.

Additional Sessions Requested to Complete Treatment: 2

Comparative Analysis of the Two Treatment Update Requests

There are a number of problems with the first treatment update request: The therapist's treatment goal was too vague, was not negotiated in behavioral terms, and was too monolithic. As therapists we can never be absolutely certain why a child behaves in a particular way. The treatment approach being used by the therapist is not efficient and is more growth-oriented. Most major managed care companies do not pay for growth-oriented treatment. Rather than putting the parents in charge of solving their son's problem, the therapist has taken on this task, which is limiting in terms of potential avenues for intervention. Finally, the 20 therapy visits requested by the therapist would automatically close the negotiation door with any case manager. Many clients who have managed health plans are only allotted 20 to 30 mental health visits per calendar year. Therefore, a case manager will prevent any therapist from exhausting all their client's benefits.

The second report is characterized by well-formed and solvable behavioral goals and a realistic treatment plan. The treatment approach the therapist is using is time-sensitive, action-oriented, and managed care friendly. Within six sessions, the therapist has helped the family achieve their goals. At the beginning of treatment this therapist also recognized the importance of actively collaborating with Stephen's teacher, who was both the referring person and key member of the problem system.

CONCLUSION

In this chapter, I have presented many practical guidelines for empowering families and therapists in the world of managed care. By following the guidelines offered in this chapter, therapists will increase their marketability to managed care companies, increase their referrals, and provide more focused and goal-oriented treatment with children and their families. As managed care is here to stay, why not make it work for you!

CHAPTER 10

Solution-Focused Therapy and Beyond: Major Themes and Implications for the Future

Unless you try to do something beyond what you have already mastered, you will never grow.
                                    –RALPH WALDO EMERSON

MAJOR THEMES OF THE BOOK

Throughout this book, I have presented many cutting-edge theoretical ideas and therapeutic strategies that can increase our clinical effectiveness when working with challenging children and their families. At this point, I will review and summarize some of the major ideas discussed in the book and follow with a brief discussion of the implications of these therapeutic ideas for the future.

I have presented several ways to expand the basic Solution-Focused Brief Therapy model to make it more flexible and to build in more therapeutic options once clinicians have exhausted all the possibilities with the basic model. By expanding the basic model, therapists will have multiple pathways they can pursue for producing therapeutic changes with more chronic and challenging child cases.

One major therapeutic component I have added to the basic Solution-Focused Brief Therapy approach is the use of family play and art therapy tasks. By incorporating family play and art therapy techniques as one possible therapeutic pathway to pursue with children, we can gain access to the children's intrapsychic worlds and capitalize on the natural ways children best express themselves. As shown in the case examples presented throughout this book, the play and art activity of children can serve as the catalyst for altering their parents' unhelpful beliefs about them and problem-maintaining parent–child interactions. By using play and art techniques with children and their families, we are also breaking down the barriers that have divided child and family therapists for decades.

A good grasp of child development, particularly what a child is capable of cognitively understanding, feeling, and mastering behaviorally at any stage of development, can inform how we interview the child and what we choose to do with task design and selection. By having this knowledge base, therapists can educate parents on what to expect at a given stage of development and normalize for parents child behaviors that typically occur at a particular age or in response to family life-cycle changes.

Throughout this book, I have stressed the importance of empowering children by giving them a "voice" in their own treatment and in their own lives. Too often, therapists working with children concentrate most of their therapeutic efforts on intervening through the child's parents and tend to act as the child's mouthpiece at collaborative meetings with school personnel or other involved helpers from larger systems. Rarely do family therapists, or brief therapists for that matter invite their child clients to identify their goals, nor do they advocate for the children to edit or offer a rebuttal to the school psychologist's case study evaluation report or to have a say in future school planning. Often, mental health professionals and parents forget that children are people too and should be given the respect and freedom to be active advisers on their own lives.

The research on resilient children has identified several key protective factors that clinicians should attempt to identify, accentuate, and capitalize on in their problem-solving efforts with their child clients and their families. Many of the findings from these research studies have challenged widely held beliefs by social scientists and mental health professionals that children with a mentally ill, chemically impaired, or abusive parent will grow up to be emotionally and socially handicapped. The results of several longitudinal studies with resilient children indicate that they grow up to become well-adjusted, optimistic, and in many cases, productive adults.

IMPLICATIONS FOR THE FUTURE

Many predict that by the year 2000, more than 50% of current private practitioners will be out of jobs as a result of the loss of fee-for-service business (Cummings, 1996). As client indemnity insurance plans are increasingly being replaced by health maintenance organizations and preferred provider organizations and fee-for-service business continues to dry up, private practitioners and agency staff will need therapeutic tools to survive and thrive in our rapidly changing health care environment. The integrative Solution-Focused Brief Therapy approach presented in this book is managed care friendly and provides clinicians with the therapeutic armamentaria to do effective short-term work with children and their families. Managed care companies are constantly looking for therapists who work briefly with children and their families (Poynter, 1994). Therefore, expertise in providing Solution-Focused Therapy with children will make a therapist highly marketable to major managed care companies.

Garmezy (1971) has referred to resilient children as "the children of the dream" (p. 114). Resilient children have taught researchers a great deal about how to persevere and cope with growing up in high-stress family and social environments. The children's stories describe a combination of individual, familial, and social factors that had a steeling effect on them and empowered them to overcome adversity. Clinicians should familiarize themselves with these key protective factors and inquire with children and their parents about their past successes at overcoming adverse life events and how the child manages stressful situations and explore whether any of these protective factors are present and can be harnessed to help resolve the current presenting problems. Primary- and secondary-prevention psychoeducational groups can be conducted for children identified as high risk. In such groups children can learn how to identify, enhance, and develop the coping skills to become resilient children. I have also developed a Solution-Oriented Parenting Group model (Selekman, 1993) for parents of adolescents, which can also be used with parents of younger children and can teach them the importance of maintaining an optimistic parental stance, how to capitalize on their past parental problem-solving successes, and how to accentuate their children's strengths.

In this book, I have presented an integrative Solution-Focused Brief Therapy approach for children and their families. The model is competency-based and collaborative and invites families to define the goals for treatment. A unique feature to this model is the use of children as expert consultants to their parents, to the therapist, and to involved helping professionals from larger systems. Children make excellent shamans. They can heal their parents in ways that therapists can never replicate. It is my hope that the therapeutic ideas discussed in this book will help therapists find the creative edge in their work, inject more playfulness into their sessions, and provide them with the therapeutic tools to do effective and efficient clinical work with children and their families.

References

Achenbach, T. (1990). Conceptualization of developmental psychopathology. In M. Lewis & S. M. Miller (Eds.), *Handbook of developmental psychopathology* (pp. 3–14). New York: Plenum Press.

Allgood, S. M., Parham, K. B., Salts, C. J., & Smith, T. A. (1995). The association between pretreatment change and unplanned termination in family therapy. *American Journal of Family Therapy, 23*(3), 195–202.

American Psychiatric Association. (1994). *Diagnostic and statistical manual of mental disorders* (4th ed.). Washington, DC: Author.

Andersen, T. (1991). *The reflecting team: Dialogues and dialogues about the dialogues.* New York: Norton.

Andersen, T. (1995). Reflecting processes; acts of informing and forming: You can borrow my eyes, but you must not take them away from me. In S. Friedman (Ed.), *The reflecting team in action: Collaborative practice in family therapy* (pp. 11–38). New York: Guilford Press.

Anderson, H. (1996). A reflection on client-professional collaboration. *Family Systems and Health, 14*(2), 193–203.

Anderson, H., & Goolishian, H. (1988a). *Changing thoughts on self, agency, questions, narrative and therapy.* Unpublished manuscript.

Anderson, H., & Goolishian, H. (1988b). Human systems as linguistic systems: Preliminary and evolving ideas about the implications for clinical theory. *Family Process, 27*(4), 371–395.

Anderson, H., & Goolishian, H. (1991a, October). *"Not knowing": A critical element of a collaborative language systems therapy approach.* Plenary address presented at the annual conference of the American Association for Marriage and Family Therapy, Dallas, TX.

Anderson, H., & Goolishian, H. (1991b). Thinking about multiagency work with substance abusers and their families: A language systems approach. *Journal of Strategic and Systemic Therapies, 10*(1), 20–36.

Anthony, E. J. (1984). The St. Louis risk research project. In N. F. Watt, E. J. Anthony, L. C. Wynne, & J. Roth (Eds.), *Children at risk for schizophrenia: A longitudinal perspective* (pp. 105–148). Cambridge, UK: Cambridge University Press.

Anthony, E. J. (1987). Risk, vulnerability, and resilience: An overview. In E. J. Anthony & B. J. Cohler (Eds.), *The invulnerable child* (pp. 3–48). New York: Guilford Press.

Anthony, E. J., & Cohler, B. J. (Eds.). (1987). *The invulnerable child.* New York: Guilford Press.

Avis, J. M. (1986). Feminist issues in family therapy. In F. P. Piercy, D. H. Sprenkle, and Associates, *Family therapy sourcebook* (pp. 213–243). New York: Guilford Press.

Barkley, R. A. (1995). *Taking charge of ADHD: The complete, authoritative guide for parents.* New York: Guilford Press.

Barkley, R. A., Guevremont, D. C., Anastopoulos, A. D., & Fletcher, K. F. (1992). A comparison of three family therapy programs for treating family conflicts in adolescents with ADHD. *Journal of Consulting and Clinical Psychology, 60,* 450–462.

Barrett, T. H. (1993). *Tao: To know and not be knowing.* San Francisco: Chronicle Books.

Berg, I. K., & de Shazer, S. (1991). Solution talk. In D. Sollee (Ed.), *Constructing the future* (pp. 15–29). Washington, DC: American Association for Marriage and Family Therapy.

Berg, I. K., & de Shazer, S. (1993). Making numbers talk: Language in therapy. In S. Friedman (Ed.), *The new language of change: Constructive collaboration in psychotherapy* (pp. 5–24). New York: Guilford Press.

Berg, I. K., & Gallagher, D. (1991). Solution-focused brief treatment with adolescent substance abusers. In T. C. Todd & M. D. Selekman (Eds.), *Family therapy approaches with adolescent substance abusers* (pp. 93–111). Needham Heights, MA: Allyn & Bacon.

Berg, I. K., & Miller, S. D. (1992). *Working with the problem drinker: A solution-focused approach.* New York: Norton.

Bleuler, M. (1978). *The schizophrenic disorders.* New Haven, CT: Yale University Press.

Bloom, B. L. (1981). Focused single-session therapy: Initial development and evaluation. In S. H. Budman (Ed.), *Forms of brief therapy* (pp. 167–216). New York: Guilford Press.

Bogdan, J. (1984). Family organization as an ecology of ideas. *Family Process, 23,* 375–388.

Bogdan, J. (1986, July/August). Do families really need problems? Why am I not a functionalist. *Family Therapy Networker,* pp. 31–69.

Bograd, M. (1990). Scapegoating mothers: Conceptual errors in systems formulations. In M. P. Mirkin (Ed.), *The social and political contexts of family therapy* (pp. 69–89). Needham Heights, MA: Allyn & Bacon.

Bohm, D. (1985). *Unfolding meaning.* Loveland, CO: Foundation House.

Bohm, D. (1996). *On dialogue.* London: Routledge.

Bonny, H. L., & Savary, L. M. (1973). *Music and your mind.* New York: Harper & Row.

Briggs, J. (1992). *Fractals: The patterns of chaos.* New York: Simon & Schuster.

Brookfield, S. D. (1987). *Developing critical thinkers.* San Francisco, CA: Jossey-Bass.

Brown, J., & Isaacs, D. (1997). Conversation as a core business process. *The System's Thinker, 7*(10), 1–6.

Browning, C. H. (1996). Practice survival strategies: Business basics for effective marketing to managed care. In N. A. Cummings, M. S. Pallak, & J. L. Cummings (Eds.), *Surviving the demise of solo practice: Mental health practitioners prospering in the era of managed care* (pp. 145–174). Madison, CT: Psychosocial Press.

Buzan, T. (1984). *Make the most of your mind.* New York: Fireside.

Buzan, T. (1989). *Use both sides of your brain.* New York: Penguin Books.

Campbell, T. W. (1996). Systemic therapies and basic research. *Journal of Systemic Therapies, 15*(3), 15–40.

Capra, F. (1988). *Uncommon wisdom: Conversations with remarkable people.* New York: Bantam Books.

Carter, B., & McGoldrick, M. (1988). *The changing family life cycle: A framework for family therapy.* New York: Gardner Press.

Casement, P. J. (1985). *Learning from the patient.* New York: Guilford Press.

Ceci, S. J., Ross, D. F., & Toglia, M. P. (1987). Age differences in suggestibility: Narrowing and uncertainties. In S. J. Ceci, M. P. Toglia, & D. F. Ross (Eds.), *Children's eyewitness memory* (pp. 79–91). New York: Springer-Verlag.

Chang, J., & Phillips, M. (1993). Michael White and Steve de Shazer: New directions in family therapy. In S. Gilligan & R. Price (Eds.), *Therapeutic conversations* (pp. 95–112). New York: Norton.

Chodron, P. (1994). *Start where you are: A guide to compassionate living.* Boston: Shambhala.

Cole, C. B., & Loftus, E. F. (1987). The memory of children. In S. J. Ceci, M. P. Toglia, & D. F. Ross (Eds.), *Children's eyewitness memory* (pp. 178–208). New York: Springer-Verlag.

Cooperrider, D. L., Svivastva, S. (1987). Appreciative inquiry in organizational life. *Research in Organizational Change and Development, 1,* 129–169.

Cottrell, L. S., & Foote, N. N. (1995). Sullivan's contributions to social psychology. In P. Mullahy (Ed.), *The contributions of Harry Stack Sullivan* (pp. 181–207). Northvale, NJ: Jason Aronson.

Cowan, P. A. (1978). *Piaget with feeling: Cognitive, social, and emotional dimensions.* New York: Holt, Rinehart & Winston.

Cowen, E. L., Pedersen, A., Babigian, H., Izzo, L. D., & Trost, M. A. (1973). Long-term follow-up of early detected vulnerable children. *Journal of Consulting and Clinical Psychology, 41,* 438–446.

Csikszentmihalyi, M., & Getzels, J. W. (1970). Concern for discovery: An attitudinal component of creative production. *Journal of Personality, 38*(1), 91–105.

Cummings, N. A. (1996). The impact of managed care employment and training: A primer for survival. In N. A. Cummings, M. S. Pallak, & J. L.

Cummings (Eds.), *Surviving the demise of solo practice: Mental health practitioners prospering in the era of managed care* (pp. 11–26). Madison, CT: Psychosocial Press.

Daehler, M. W., & Greco, C. (1985). Memory in very young children. In M. Pressley & C. J. Brainerd (Eds.), *Cognitive learning and memory in children* (pp. 92–117). New York: Springer-Verlag.

Dawes, R. M. (1994). *House of cards: Psychology and psychotherapy built on myth.* New York: Free Press.

DeBono, E. (1992). *Serious creativity.* New York: HarperCollins.

de Shazer, S. (1985). *Keys to solution in brief therapy.* New York: Norton.

de Shazer, S. (1988). *Clues: Investigating solutions in brief therapy.* New York: Norton.

de Shazer, S. (1991). *Putting difference to work.* New York: Norton.

de Shazer, S. (1994). *Words were originally magic.* New York: Norton.

de Shazer, S., & White, M. (1996, October). *Narrative solutions/solution narratives.* Conference sponsored by the Brief Therapy Center, Milwaukee, WI.

Diener, C. I., & Dweck, C. S. (1978). An analysis of learned helplessness: Continuous changes in performance, strategy, and achievement cognitions following failure. *Journal of Personality and Social Psychology, 36,* 451–462.

DiLeo, J. H. (1973). *Children's drawings as diagnostic aids.* New York: Brunner/Mazel.

Dillon, J. T. (1992). Problem-finding and solving. In S. J. Parnes (Ed.), *Sourcebook for creative problem-solving* (pp. 305–314). Buffalo, NY: Creative Education Foundation Press.

Dilts, R. B. (1994). *Strategies of genius* (Vol. II). Cupertino, CA: Meta.

Dinkmeyer, D., & McKay, G. D. (1989). *The parent's handbook.* Circle Pines, MN: American Guidance Service.

Doherty, W. J. (1995). The whys and levels of collaborative family healthcare. *Family Systems Medicine, 13*(3/4), 275–283.

Durrant, M., & Coles, D. (1991). The Michael White approach. In T. C. Todd & M. D. Selekman (Eds.), *Family therapy approaches with adolescent substance abusers* (pp. 135–175). Needham Heights, MA: Allyn & Bacon.

Dweck, C. S. (1975). The role of expectations and attributions in the alleviation of learned helplessness. *Journal of Personality and Social Psychology, 31,* 674–685.

Eastwood, M., Sweeney, D., & Piercy, F. (1987). The "no-problem problem": A family therapy approach for certain first-time adolescent substance abusers. *Family Relations, 36,* 125–128.

Epston, D. (1989). *The collected papers of David Epston.* Adelaide, South Australia: Dulwich Centre Publications.

Erickson, M. H., & Havens, R. A. (1985). *The wisdom of Milton H. Erickson: Human behavior and psychotherapy* (Vol. II). New York: Irvington.

Erickson, M. H., & Rossi, E. (1983). *Healing in hypnosis.* New York: Irvington Publishers.

Festinger, T. (1983). *No one ever asked us.* New York: Columbia University Press.

Forehand, R., & Long, N. (1996). *Parenting the strong-willed child.* Chicago: Contemporary Books.

Fraser, J. S. (1995). Process, problems, and solutions in brief therapy. *Journal of Marital and Family Therapy, 21*(3), 265–279.

Freeman, J. C., & Lobovits, D. (1993). The turtle with wings. In S. Friedman (Ed.), *The new language of change: Constructive collaboration in psychotherapy* (pp. 188–226). New York: Guilford Press.

Fruggeri, L. (1992). Therapeutic process as the social construction of change. In S. McNamee & K. J. Gergen (Eds.), *Therapy as a social construction* (pp. 40–54). London: Sage.

Gabarino, J., & Stott, F. M. (1992). *What children can tell us: Eliciting, interpreting, and evaluating critical information from children.* San Francisco: Jossey-Bass.

Garmezy, N. (1971). Vulnerability research and the issue of primary prevention. *American Journal of Orthopsychiatry, 41*(1), 101–116.

Garmezy, N. (1981). Children under stress: Perspectives on antecedents and correlates of vulnerability and resistance to psychopathology. In A. I. Rabin, J. Aronoff, A. M. Barclay, & R. Zucker (Eds.), *Further explorations in personality* (pp. 101–116). New York: Wiley.

Garmezy, N. (1991). Resiliency and vulnerability to adverse developmental outcomes associated with poverty. *American Behavioral Scientist, 34,* 416–430.

Garmezy, N. (1993). Children in poverty: Resilience despite risk. In D. Reiss, J. E. Richters, M. Radke-Yarrow, & D. Scharff (Eds.), *Children and violence* (pp. 127–136). New York: Guilford Press.

Garmezy, N. (1994). Reflections and commentary on risk, resilience, and development. In R. J. Haggerty, L. R. Sherrod, N. Garmezy, & M. Rutter (Eds.), *Stress, risk, and resilience in children and adolescents: Processes, mechanisms, and in interventions* (pp. 1–19). Cambridge, UK: Cambridge University Press.

Gauron, E. F., & Dickson, J. K. (1969). The influence of seeing the patient first on diagnostic decision-making in psychiatry. *American Journal of Psychiatry, 126,* 199–205.

Gelb, M. J. (1995). *Thinking for a change.* New York: Harmony Books.

Getzels, J. W. (1992). Problem-finding and the inventiveness of solutions. In S. J. Parnes (Ed.), *Sourcebook for creative problem-solving* (pp. 301–305). Buffalo, NY: Creative Education Foundation Press.

Getzels, J. W., & Csikszentmihalyi, M. (1976a). From problem-solving to problem-finding. In I. A. Taylor & J. W. Getzels (Eds.), *Perspectives in creativity* (pp. 240–267). Chicago: Aldine.

Getzels, J. W., & Csikszentmihalyi, M. (1976b). *The creative vision: A longitudinal study of problem-finding in art.* New York: Wiley.

Gil, E. (1994). *Play in family therapy.* New York: Guilford Press.

Gingerich, W., & de Shazer, S. (1991). The BRIEFER project: Using expert systems as theory construction tools. *Family Process, 30,* 241–249.

Gingerich, W. J., de Shazer, S., & Weiner-Davis, M. (1988). Constructing change: A research view of interviewing. In E. Lipchik (Ed.), *Interviewing* (pp. 21–31). Rockville, MD: Aspen.

Goodrich, T. J. (1991). Women, power, and family therapy: What's wrong with this picture? *Journal of Feminist Family Therapy, 3*(1/2), 5–38.

Goolishian, H. (1990). Family therapy: An evolving story. *Contemporary Family Therapy, 12*(3), 173–180.

Gordon, D., & Meyers-Anderson, M. (1981). *Phoenix: Therapeutic patterns of Milton H. Erickson.* Cupertino, CA: Meta.

Gordon, T. (1970). *P.E.T.: Parent effectiveness training.* New York: Plume.

Gordon, W. J. (1992). On being explicit about creative process. In S. J. Parnes (Ed.), *Sourcebook for creative problem-solving* (pp. 164–168). Buffalo, NY: Creative Education Foundation Press.

Gordon, W. J., & Poze, T. (1981). Conscious/subconscious interaction in a creative act. *Journal of Creative Behavior, 15*(1), 55–65.

Greenspan, S. I. (1995). *The challenging child: Understanding, raising, and enjoying the five "difficult" types of children.* Reading, MA: Addison-Wesley.

Haggerty, R. J., Sherrod, L. R., Garmezy, N., & Rutter, M. (1994). *Stress, risk, and resilience in children and adolescents: Processes, mechanisms, and interventions.* Cambridge, UK: Cambridge University Press.

Haley, J. (1986). *Uncommon therapy: The psychiatric techniques of Milton H. Erickson, M.D.* (2nd ed.). New York: Norton.

Haley, J. (1987). *Problem-solving therapy* (2nd ed.). San Francisco: Jossey-Bass.

Hiatt, D., & Hargrave, G. E. (1995, July/August). The characteristics of highly effective therapists in managed behavioral provider networks. *Behavioral Healthcare Tomorrow,* pp. 19–22.

Hoffman, L. (1990). Constructing realities: An art of lenses. *Family Process, 29,* 1–12.

Howard, K. L., Kopta, S. M., Krause, M. S., & Orlinsky, D. E. (1986). The dose–effect relationship in psychotherapy. *American Psychologist, 41,* 159–164.

Isaacs, W. (1993). Dialogue: The power of collective thinking. *The Systems Thinker, 4*(3), 1–4.

Jansson, T. (1962). *Moomin's invisible friend.* London: Heinemann.

Jenkins, A. (1994). Therapy for abuse or therapy as abuse? *Dulwich Centre Newsletter, 1,* 11–19.

Johnson, L. N., & Nelson, T. S. (1996, October). *Noticing pretreatment change and therapeutic outcome.* Poster session presented at the annual conference of the American Association for Marriage and Family Therapy, Toronto, Ontario, Canada.

Kabat-Zinn, J. (1994). *Wherever you go there you are: Mindfulness meditation in everyday life.* New York: Hyperion.

Kauffman, C., Grunebaum, H., Cohler, B., & Gamer, E. (1979). Superkids: Competent children of psychotic mothers. *American Journal of Psychiatry, 136,* 1398–1402.

Keith, D. V., & Whitaker, C. A. (1994). Play therapy: A paradigm for work with families. In C. Schaefer & L. Carey (Eds.), *Family play therapy* (pp. 185–202). Northvale, NJ: Jason Aronson.

Kohut, H. (1971). *The analysis of the self.* New York: International Universities Press.

Kwiatkowska, H. Y. (1978). *Family therapy and evaluation through art.* Springfield, IL: Charles C Thomas.

Landau-Stanton, J. (1990). Issues of methods of treatment for families in cultural transition. In M. P. Mirkin (Ed.), *The social and political contexts of family therapy* (pp. 251–275). Needham Heights, MA: Allyn & Bacon.

Leake, G. J., & King, A. S. (1977). Effect of counselor expectations on alcoholic recovery. *Alcohol Health and Research World, 1*(3), 16–22.

Lebow, J., & Gurman, A. S. (1996, January/February). Making a difference: A new research review offers good news to couples and family therapists. *Family Therapy Networker,* pp. 69–76.

Levin, R. (1987). Liner notes for *Outward bound: The music of the Eric Dolphy quintet.* Prestige/New Jazz 8236.

Lipchik, E. (1988). Purposeful sequences for beginning the solution-focused interview. In E. Lipchik (Ed.), *Interviewing* (pp. 105–116). Rockville, MD: Aspen.

Luepnitz, D. (1988). *The family interpreted.* New York: Basic Books.

Mackworth, N. H. (1965). Originality. *American Psychologist, 20,* 51–66.

Madanes, C. (1981). *Strategic family therapy.* San Francisco: Jossey-Bass.

Masten, A., Best, K. M., & Garmezy, N. (1990). Resilience and development: Contributions from the study of children who overcome adversity. *Development and Psychopathology, 2,* 425–444.

Masten, A., & Garmezy, N. (1985). Risk, vulnerability, and protective factors in developmental psychopathology. In B. B. Lahey & A. E. Kazdin (Eds.), *Advances in clinical child psychology* (pp. 1–52). New York: Plenum Press.

McDaniel, S. H., Campbell, T. L., & Seaburn, D. B. (1995). Principles for collaboration between health and mental health providers in primary care. *Family Systems Medicine, 13*(3/4), 283–299.

McLuhan, M. (1964). *Understanding the media: The extensions of man.* New York: McGraw-Hill.

Miller, S. D., & Berg, I. K. (1995). *The miracle method: A radically new approach to problem drinking.* New York: Norton.

Minuchin, S. (1974). *Families and family therapy.* Cambridge, MA: Harvard University Press.

Mitchell, S. (1988). *Tao Te Ching: A new English version.* New York: HarperCollins.

Moore, M. T. (1985). The relationship between the originality of essays and variables in the problem-discovery process: A study of creative and non-creative middle school students. *Research in the Teaching of English, 19*(1), 84–95.

Moskovitz, S. (1983). *Love despite hate.* New York: Schocken Books.

Newfield, N. A., Kuehl, B. P., Joanning, H. P., & Quinn, W. H. (1991). We can tell you about "psychos" and "shrinks": An ethnography of the family therapy of adolescent drug abuse. In T. C. Todd & M. D. Selekman (Eds.), *Family therapy approaches with adolescent substance abusers* (pp. 275–307). Needham Heights, MA: Allyn & Bacon.

Nichols, M. P. (1995). *The lost art of listening.* New York: Guilford Press.

Nisker, W. S. (1990). *Crazy wisdom.* Berkeley, CA: Ten Speed.

O'Hanlon, W. H. (1987). *Taproots: Underlying principles of Milton Erickson's therapy and hypnosis.* New York: Norton.

O'Hanlon, W. H., & Weiner-Davis, M. (1989). *In search of solutions: A new direction in psychotherapy.* New York: Norton.

Osborn, A. F. (1993). *Applied imagination: Principles and procedures of creative problem-solving* (3rd ed.). Buffalo, NY: Creative Education Foundation Press.

Oss, M. E., & Stair, T. (1996). *Managed behavioral health market share in the United States 1996–1997.* Gettysburg, PA: Behavioral Health Industry News.

Oster, G. D., & Gould, P. (1987). *Using drawings in assessment and therapy.* New York: Brunner/Mazel.

Ostrander, S., Schroeder, L., & Ostrander, N. (1994). *Superlearning 2000.* New York: Dell.

Palazzoli, M. S., Boscolo, L., Cecchin, G., & Prata, G. (1980). Hypothesizing—circularity—neutrality: Three guidelines for the conductor of the session. *Family Process, 19*(1), 3–13.

Palmarini, M. P. (1994). *Inevitable illusions: How mistakes of reason rule our minds.* New York: Wiley.

Parnes, S. J. (1992). *Visionizing.* Buffalo, NY: Creative Education Foundation Press.

Peek, C. J., & Heinrich, R. L. (1995). Building a collaborative healthcare organization: From idea to invention to innovation. *Family Systems Medicine, 13*(3/4), 327–343.

Phillips, J. (1986, May/June). Language, communication, and the therapeutic context: A review. *Family Therapy Newsletter,* pp. 5–7.

Pinderhughes, E. (1990). Legacy of slavery: The experience of black families in America. In M. P. Mirkin (Ed.), *The social and political contexts of family therapy* (pp. 289–305). Needham Heights, MA: Allyn & Bacon.

Poynter, W. L. (1994). *The preferred provider's handbook: Building a successful private therapy practice in the managed care marketplace.* New York: Brunner/Mazel.

Prince, G. M. (1992). The mindspring theory: A new development from synectics research. In S. J. Parnes (Ed.), *Sourcebook for creative problem-solving* (pp. 177–193). Buffalo, NY: Creative Education Foundation Press.

Prochaska, J. O., Norcross, J. C., & DiClemente, C. C. (1994). *Changing for good.* New York: Morrow.

Rhyne, J. (1996). *The gestalt art experience: Patterns that connect*. Chicago: Magnolia Street.

Riley, S., & Malchiodi, C. A. (1994). *Integrative approaches to family art therapy*. Chicago: Magnolia Street.

Rinpoche, L. Z. (1993). *Transforming problems into happiness*. Boston: Wisdom.

Rokeach, M. (1950). The effect of perception time upon rigidity and concreteness of thinking. *Journal of Experimental Psychology, 40*, 206–216.

Rosemond, J. (1994). *Daily guide to parenting*. Marshaltown, IA: Thoughtful Books.

Rubin, Z. (1980). *Children's friendships*. Cambridge, MA: Harvard University Press.

Salamon, E., & Grevelius, K. (1996, June). *Who has got a problem with what?: Why social workers and therapists in Sweden have got a drinking problem*. A workshop presented at the conference on NLP and other Solution-Oriented Approaches, Jyvaskyla, Finland.

Saywitz, K. (1987). Children's testimony: Age-related patterns of memory errors. In S. J. Ceci, M. P. Toglia, & D. F. Ross (Eds.), *Children's eyewitness memory* (pp. 33–52). New York: Springer-Verlag.

Schaefer, C. E., & DiGeronimo, T. F. (1995, February). Making sense of make-believe: Understanding and encouraging your child's imagination. *Child*, pp. 29–33.

Schafer, R. (1980). *Narrative actions in psychoanalysis*. Worcester, MA: Clark University Press.

Schon, D. A. (1983). *The reflective practitioner: How professionals think in action*. New York: Basic Books.

Schrage, M. (1990). *Shared minds: The new technologies of collaboration*. New York: Random House.

Selekman, M. D. (1991). "With a little help from my friends": The use of peers in the family therapy of adolescent substance abusers. *Family Dynamics of Addiction Quarterly, 1*(1), 69–77.

Selekman, M. D. (1993). *Pathways to change: Brief therapy solutions with difficult adolescents*. New York: Guilford Press.

Selekman, M. D. (1995a). "Help me out . . . I'm confused": The Columbo approach with difficult youth. *Newsletter of the Brief Therapy Network, 1*(4), 1–4.

Selekman, M. D. (1995b). Rap music with wisdom: Peer reflecting teams with tough adolescents. In S. Friedman (Ed.), *The reflecting team in action: Collaborative practice in family therapy* (pp. 205–223). New York: Guilford Press.

Selekman, M. D. (1996). Turning out the light on a seasonal affective disorder. *Journal of Systemic Therapies, 15*(3), 40–51.

Seligman, M. E. (1995). *The optimistic child: A revolutionary program that safeguards children against depression and builds lifelong resilience*. Boston: Houghton-Mifflin.

Senge, P. M., Kleiner, A., Roberts, C., Ross, R. B., & Smith, B. J. (1994). *The fifth discipline fieldbook: Strategies and tools for building a learning organization*. New York: Currency and Doubleday.

Seuss, D. (1961a). *The Sneetches.* New York: Random House.

Seuss, D. (1961b). *The Zax.* New York: Random House.

Sluzki, C. E. (1979). Migration and family conflict. *Family Process, 18*(4), 379–390.

Sobol, B. (1982). Art therapy and strategic family therapy. *American Journal of Art Therapy, 21,* 23–31.

Spence, D. (1982). *Narrative truth and historical truth.* New York: Norton.

Stith, S. M., Rosen, K. H., McCollum, E. E., Coleman, J. U., & Herman, S. A. (1996). The voices of children: Preadolescent children's experiences in family therapy. *Journal of Marital and Family Therapy, 22*(1), 69–86.

Taffel, R. (1991). *Parenting by heart.* Reading, MA: Addison-Wesley.

Talmon, M. (1990). *Single session therapy.* San Francisco: Jossey-Bass.

Thomas, E., Polansky, N., & Kounin, J. (1955). The expected behavior of a potentially helpful person. *Human Relations, 8,* 165–174.

Tinnin, L. (1990). Biological processes in nonverbal communication and their role in the making and interpretations of art. *American Journal of Art Therapy, 29,* 9–13.

Tomm, K. (1987). Interventive interviewing: Part II. Reflexive questioning as a means to enable self-healing. *Family Process, 26,* 167–183.

Tomm, K., & White, M. (1987, October). *Externalizing problems and internalizing directional choices.* Training Institute presented at the annual conference of the American Association for Marriage and Family Therapy, Chicago.

Trepper, T. S., & Barrett, M. J. (1989). *Systemic treatment of incest.* New York: Brunner/Mazel.

Vandenberg, J. (1993). Integration of individualized mental health services into the system of care for children and adolescents. *Administration and Policy in Mental Health, 20*(4), 91–112.

Van Gundy, A. B. (1988). *Stalking the wild solution: A problem-finding approach to creative problem-solving.* Buffalo, NY: Bearly Limited.

Van Gundy, A. B. (1992). *Idea power.* New York: AMACOM.

Wachtel, E. F. (1994). *Treating troubled children and their families.* New York: Guilford Press.

Walsh, F., & Scheinkman, M. (1989). Female: The hidden gender dimension in models of family therapy. In M. McGoldrick, C. M. Andersen, & F. Walsh (Eds.), *Women in families: A framework for family therapy* (pp. 16–42). New York: Norton.

Watzlawick, P., Weakland, J., & Fisch, R. (1974). *Change: Principles of problem formation and problem resolution.* New York: Norton.

Weiner-Davis, M., de Shazer, S., & Gingerich, W. (1987). Building on pretreatment change to construct the therapeutic solution: An exploratory study. *Journal of Marital and Family Therapy, 13*(4), 359–363.

Wenger, W. (1985). *A method of personal growth and development.* Gaithersburg, MD: Psychogenics Press.

Wenger, W., & Poe, R. (1996). *The Einstein factor.* Rocklin, CA: Prima.

Werner, E. E. (1987a). Resilient children. In E. M. Hetherington & R. D. Parke (Eds.), *Contemporary readings in child psychology*. New York: McGraw-Hill.

Werner, E. E. (1987b). Vulnerability and resiliency in children at risk for delinquency: A longitudinal study from birth to young adulthood. In J. D. Burchard & S. N. Burchard (Eds.), *Prevention in delinquent behavior* (pp. 44–60). Newbury Park, CA: Sage.

Werner, E. E., & Smith, R. S. (1982). *Vulnerable but invincible*. New York: McGraw-Hill.

Werner, E. E., & Smith, R. S. (1992). *Overcoming the odds*. Ithaca, NY: Cornell University Press.

Whipple, V. (1996). Developing an identity as a feminist family therapist: Implications for training. *Journal of Marital and Family Therapy, 22*(3), 381–396.

White, M. (1988, Winter). The process of questioning: A therapy of literary merit? *Dulwich Centre Newsletter*, pp. 8–14.

White, M. (1995). *Re-authoring lives: Interviews & essays*. Adelaide, South Australia: Dulwich Centre Publications.

White, M., & Epston, D. (1990). *Narrative means to therapeutic ends*. New York: Norton.

Winnicott, D. W. (1971a). *Playing and reality*. New York: Basic Books.

Winnicott, D. W. (1971b). *Therapeutic consultations in child psychiatry*. New York: Basic Books.

Winnicott, D. W. (1985). *Deprivation and delinquency*. London: Tavistock/Routledge.

Wittgenstein, L. (1963). *On certainty*. Oxford, UK: Basil/Blackwell.

Wittgenstein, L. (1980). *Remarks on the philosophy* (Vols. I & II). Oxford, UK: Basil/Blackwell.

Wolin, S., O'Hanlon, W. H., & Hoffman, L. (1995, October). *Three strength-based therapies*. Workshop presented at the annual conference of the American Association for Marriage and Family Therapy, Baltimore.

Wolin, S. J., & Wolin, S. (1993). *The resilient self: How survivors of troubled families rise above adversity*. New York: Villard Books.

Wood, N., & Howell, F. (1993). *Spirit walker*. New York: Doubleday.

Woods, D. R. (1995, October). *Forces of change in mental health care delivery*. Plenary address at the annual conference of the Association for Marriage and Family Therapy, Baltimore.

Wujec, T. (1995). *Five star mind*. New York: Doubleday.

Yager, J. (1977). Psychiatric eclecticism: A cognitive view. *American Journal of Psychiatry, 134*, 736–741.

Zilbach, J., Bergel, E., & Gass, C. (1972). The role of young children in family therapy. In C. J. Sager & H. S. Kaplan (Eds.), *Progress in group and family therapy* (pp. 385–399). New York: Brunner/Mazel.

Index